MYNDFUL

How meditation, yoga, and mindfulness offer the keys
to living a clear, calm, and contented life.

An accessible guide for those wanting more

Dr. Ana Candia, ND

a river runs press

Published by a river runs press

978-1-7779861-0-0   MYNDFUL Hardcover book
978-1-7779861-7-9   MYNDFUL Softcover book
978-1-7779861-2-4   MYNDFUL Electronic book

Cover Design by Heather Chapman, Chapman Creative
Book Design by James Alocelja, Flocksy

Dedication

Nature! Revel in Her!

Let's consider ourselves madly lucky if we happen to live somewhere where it is safe, accessible, and socially acceptable to be outside for leisure. Nature has been, for me, a refuge, a friend, a healer, a teacher, and a reminder of the exquistely imperfect beauty this existence has to offer. Spending time outside, even if only for a short while, whether it is raining, gray, or cold, is good for our health and feelings of wellness. Studies show that proximity to nature in any form can:

- reduce depression, anxiety, and stress scores
- reduce impulsive decision making
- lower blood pressure, heart rate, cholesterol, and Type II Diabetes
- increase feelings of wellbeing and good health
- increase heart rate variability (a marker associated with recovery, resilience, and overall fitness)
- be psychologically and mentally restorative
- reduce feelings of loneliness and inadequate social support
- assist, relieve and sustain us in so, so many more ways

The research suggests these benefits are physiological effects triggered by various sensorial experiences of nature—not only via visual cues. It's pretty clear: When you aren't feeling your best, get outside. Put your phone away. Soak in the sun, the cool air, and touch something from Mother Earth. We are SO incredibly fortunate to have Her. And if you just awoke and don't even know how your day is going to go… get outside. Choose a clear and connected mind and body. MAKE it great.

To our Mother.

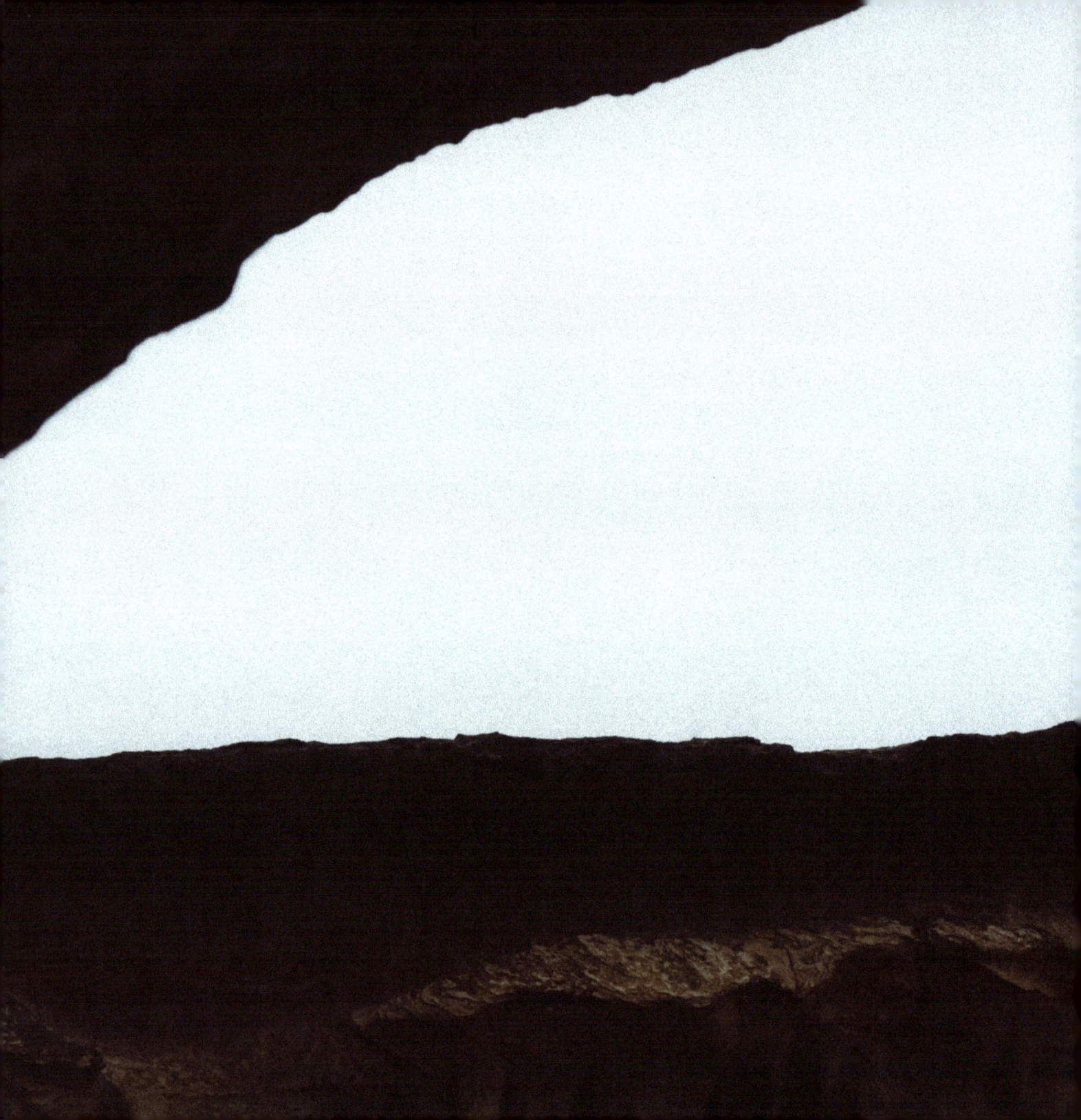

CONTENTS

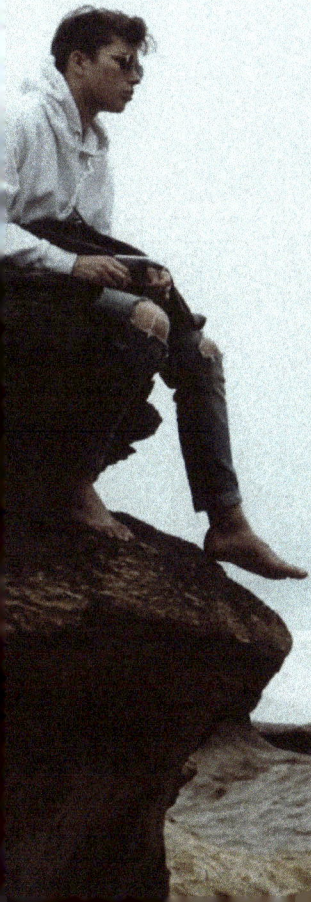

INTRODUCTION

Let me take you with me.

Have you been searching?

Or just feeling that something isn't right?

That things could feel... better than they do?

Within these pages, you will find some MYNDspace.

M – mindfulness

Y – yoga (postures, meditation, breathwork)

N – naturopathic

D – development

Here, you will encounter a space where the philosophies, central tenets, and practical teachings of the items above come together to allow you to *regain control*. To guide you to a calmer, more peaceful, more contented state of mind.

Not to worry. You don't have to practice any of these items to learn from them. But truly, as you read and become acquainted with the various teachings derived from these schools of thought, *you may find yourself actually wanting to.*

I'm sure, like me, you wouldn't appreciate anyone pushing their dogma upon you. As much as I've lived and breathed (and subsequently loved and been changed by) the practices above, you may not be familiar just yet. Or possibly you have had experience with one or more of these but wish to delve deeper.

You shouldn't have to buy cork blocks or sit cross-legged 'om'ing for hours to get close to them. Or to feel comfortable with your understanding of what they're about.

I think many people feel a sort of *that's not for me* distance with these practices. Not so much because of anything inherently off-putting or un-inviting there, but more an unintentional barrier to entry by virtue of their non-secular roots and/or a perceived esoterism they are cloaked in.

There is Sanskrit and chanting and beads and hand positions and what does it all mean, anyway? What could all of that possibly offer me if I'm not a Buddhist and I have no interest in Hindu deities?

I just want life to feel more fulfilling.

Precisely.

I wanted to write something that would remove this veil for those who are at the beginning of or still miles away from that same nudge of the gut that I had over thirteen years ago. To gently open the door and let the sun-light stream in on these ancient, profound, yet easily accessible disciplines. The guidance we glean from them has the potential to change everything for us—regardless of our religious status or belief systems.

A note on why I include naturopathic development with the other items in the grouping: When I was in school, we were taught to focus on the foun-dations of health (diet, hydration, movement, environment...) things we term "lifestyle factors." Although we are trained in and use various other modalities in our treatment plans, it's a common experience amongst na-turopathic doctors (NDs) that these lifestyle factors are the ones that cre-ate the biggest shifts in the health and wellness of our patients.

I sit across from folks every single day who, despite their primary reasons for coming to see me, are also living with overwhelm and anxiety. When these words come up and patients confirm their presence, ninety-nine times out of one hundred, we also see dysregulations in sleep, digestion, cognition, hormones, and more.

Equally ubiquitous in those with even minor anxiety is an underlying state of discontent or dissatisfaction—though usually these pieces have not registered as something to work on, to treat, or to want to resolve. For most, it's how it's always been—they don't remember a clear onset, but rather, report feeling it's been "ever since I can remember." For others, there is a known major event, trauma, or crisis that precipitated the shift and yet time, in these cases, has not healed all things.

My leanings align so well with the preponderance of scientific research supporting mindfulness, meditation, and yoga for so many conditions (namely anxiety, depression, and other mood disorders). Thus, I find myself discussing meditation apps, mindful eating techniques, and the ways that conscious breath can hack the nervous system every day, both inside and outside the clinic.

The Lifestyle Factors section on all my treatment plans is also never without notes on food and water intake, exercise, journaling, sleep routines, and getting outside. Not because of my bias, but because the copious positive studies that exist unequivocally back these as hugely effective treatment strategies for most health concerns. And when I ask patients, who a few months later are feeling a much greater sense of control over their moods and behaviors, "what do you think made the greatest difference for you?" the response I always get is, "that lifestyle stuff."

Bingo.

I've been deliberate about where I've placed emphasis here. Most people understand as a matter of logic/common sense that diet, hydration, exercise, and sleep will have some significant effects on our relative states of wellness or dis-ease. Certainly, we need help understanding exactly how to implement changes in these categories that are specific to our individual needs, histories, etc. which is why these are major conversations in any naturopathic doctor's office, mine included. The other pieces, the ones I've highlighted and tried to demystify within these pages, are the diamonds only some have unearthed.

They are not just for Buddhists or hippies or any "type" you may be imagining. These diamonds are, in fact, waiting for all of us.

MYND: It's a healing, transformative, inclusive space.
It's right here, right now, for you.

Let me help you unlearn the lie that *this is just how life feels*. Let us rip apart the myth that what's common is what's physiologically "normal."

These are the tools you've been missing.

HOW TO READ THIS BOOK

The book is comprised of six distinct sections:

LANGUAGE: Defining foundational terminology

AWARENESS: Becoming conscious, awakening

YOGA: Pose tips, tricks & takeaways, on and off the mat

MASTER TEACHERS: Wisdom from the leading authorities in this space

INSIGHTS: Perceptions with real life applications

START BY SITTING: An initiation into meditation

While each graphic-text pair works as a standalone insight or lesson, collectively they work together (in whichever order you consume them) to lift the aforementioned veil and create a sense of general understanding. You may wish to read one pair from each section daily or enjoy one section at a time. Either way, I hope that you will come back to these pages again and again as you become increasingly acquainted with the material.

In time, you will notice overlap and synergism between the disciplines. My hope is that you will find some or all of it useful and helpful in traversing your own seasons of life. If, after you've finished reading (or somewhere along the way), you have the sudden urge to roll out a mat or sign up for a meditation class, then I from-the-heart encourage you to follow that nudge as far in as it takes you.

WHY ME?

Why did I write this?

For years, I told myself I "should" be meditating. That I probably "should" take up yoga. For years I didn't get within miles of these things. All my shortness of breath and disturbed sleep and overwhelm... I was too busy studying or working or getting on with the business of the everyday that I honestly didn't connect the dots. Didn't realize those things were fixable, nor did I have any awareness that they needed fixing. I was too damned busy to notice.

One day, on a whim, I signed up for a twice weekly yoga class offered at my university. The teacher was equal parts genius and wild eccentric. There were certain positions I was pretty sure were in no yoga text ever. We also spent the first twenty to thirty minutes of each class breathing in various strange ways.

Manipulating our inhales and exhales, sending all sorts of inner dust out into the world by way of our nostrils. Pumping diaphragms like our bellies were water balloons. Hand on heart, this man would bring in newspaper clippings of athletes mid-game, extolling the virtues of their limber spines or youthful knees, placing full credit on the yoga they must be doing. Calling the classes "odd" would be something of an understatement. Certainly, they bore zero resemblance to the countless yoga classes I've since attended. Unconventional approach notwithstanding, this experience sparked a massive shift for me.

As though out of nowhere, I began sleeping restfully. Hm. I didn't realize it was sub-par to begin with. The gasps of air I would take every few breaths altogether disappeared. I felt calmer. Though we didn't seem to be doing much in the classes (no rapid heart rates or burning muscles achieved), the changes in my health and wellness were so in-my-face, I couldn't help but take notice. It got me really, really curious. So, I practiced more. When I graduated, I moved to Western Canada and decided my welcoming would be a two-week stint spent on the grounds of an ashram I knew little about. Where silent meals, meditation, yoga, and eight hours a day of physical labour were a way of life, seven days a week. There, I was introduced to concepts I had never heard of, let alone practiced or even understood.

Interest, piqued.

Craving more immersion, I spent the next year working for one of the leading yoga studios in the area. There, I had the freedom to attend all classes and, importantly, was also given constant access to the beautiful spaces between: the empty, mirrored, sun-filled rooms, the books and malas and teas, the unending conversations with a community of like-minded people, as well as an open door to monthly workshops and lectures given by master teachers from around the globe.

I worked, I practiced. I worked, I practiced.

Yoga, I soon realized, was opening a mind-body unit that didn't think itself closed. I walked as though on air.

I became acquainted with the concept of yoga "off the mat"—finding in-class/on-mat teachings so surprisingly life-applicable and useful when encountering challenges in life outside of the studio. Though I didn't have the words for it then, through breath, postures and attention, I was also cultivating present-moment awareness—this was mindfulness.

Years of practice later, I found myself contemplating a career in natural health from a compound in the Indian Himalayas, completing a 200-hour intensive Yoga Teacher Training course. Our enlightened teachers (all local swamis) lectured to us daily.

In stories and verse, they made the spectrum of human experience comprehensible, clear, and packed serenely away into the place in my brain where light shines and confusion is a long-lost stranger. To complement all the philosophical teachings, we partook in more hours of meditation, more posture and breathing classes than I care to calculate. I felt I understood....*everything*. Though of course I did not and do not, what was more important was that I had all the tools I'd ever need to make my way through this "life thing", joyfully. When the road became inevitably rocky, I had them and used them. As I do still.

I came home emboldened:
Nature and these practices were THE MEDICINE.

I studied for four more years to become licensed as a naturopathic doctor and to be able to share this medicine, in my own way, with every soul who was seeking.

Aren't we all seeking?

[A note on the photographs used in these pages:

It's quite a task, I'll admit, to choose a singular image to represent one, usually quite profound, concept. It's a task I self-imposed when I set out to create this social-media inspired, design-heavy book—a process that was as arduous as it was artistically-thrilling. In every case, I poured over hundreds of images, realizing how each would uniquely modify the concept it was supposed to represent, ultimately taking you, the reader, in varying directions. The truth is, the concepts I describe herein can be interpreted in myriad ways and they have myriad applications. But I had to make definitive choices. In some cases, they are obvious, in others, less so. I wanted to create something that was as moving visually as it was textually, and at the same time, use the images to build additional value and meaning into the in-text ideas.

Please know that I have done my utmost to fill this book with as much of the natural world as possible.

Nature. Everywhere Nature.]

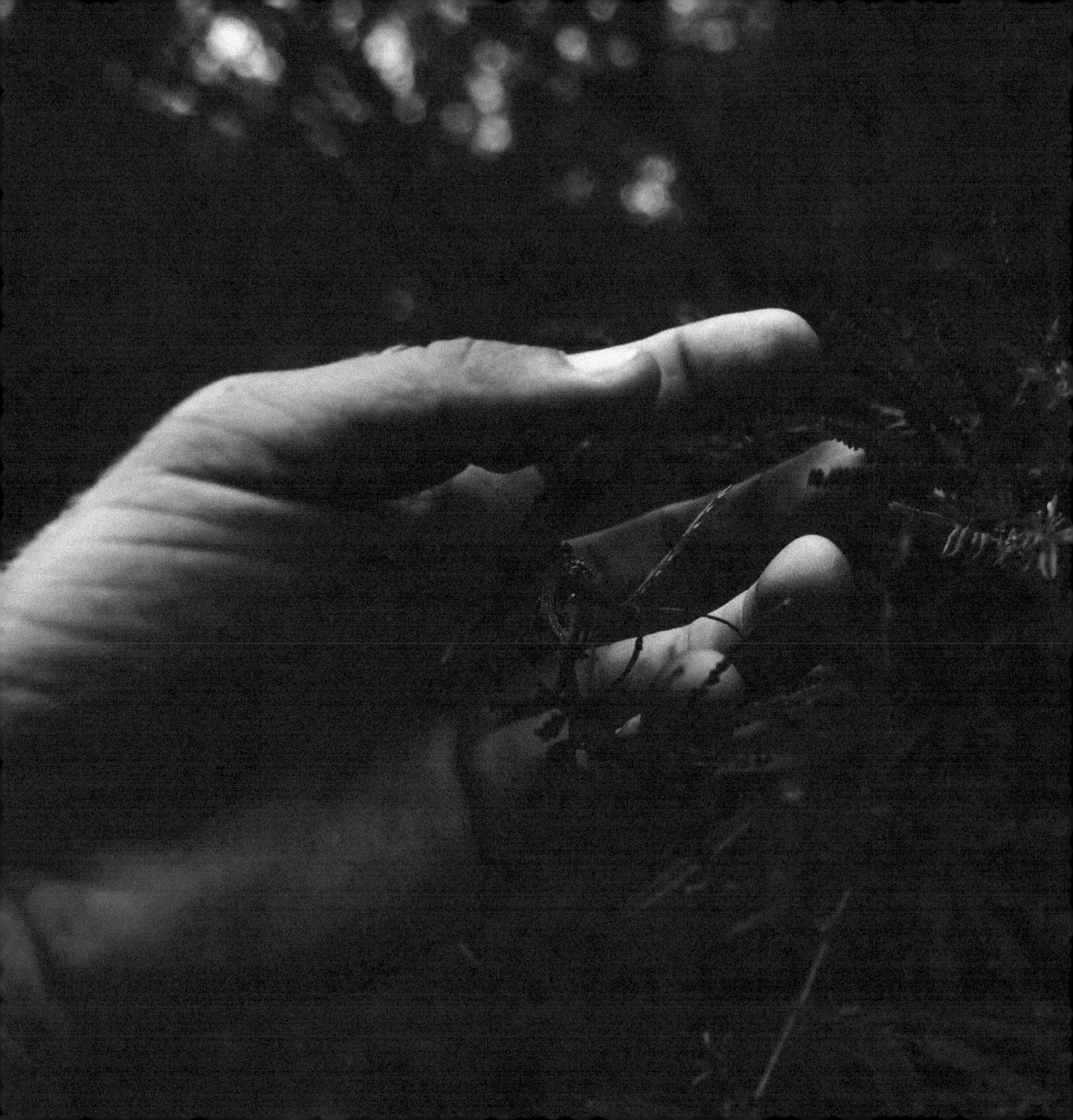

LANGUAGE

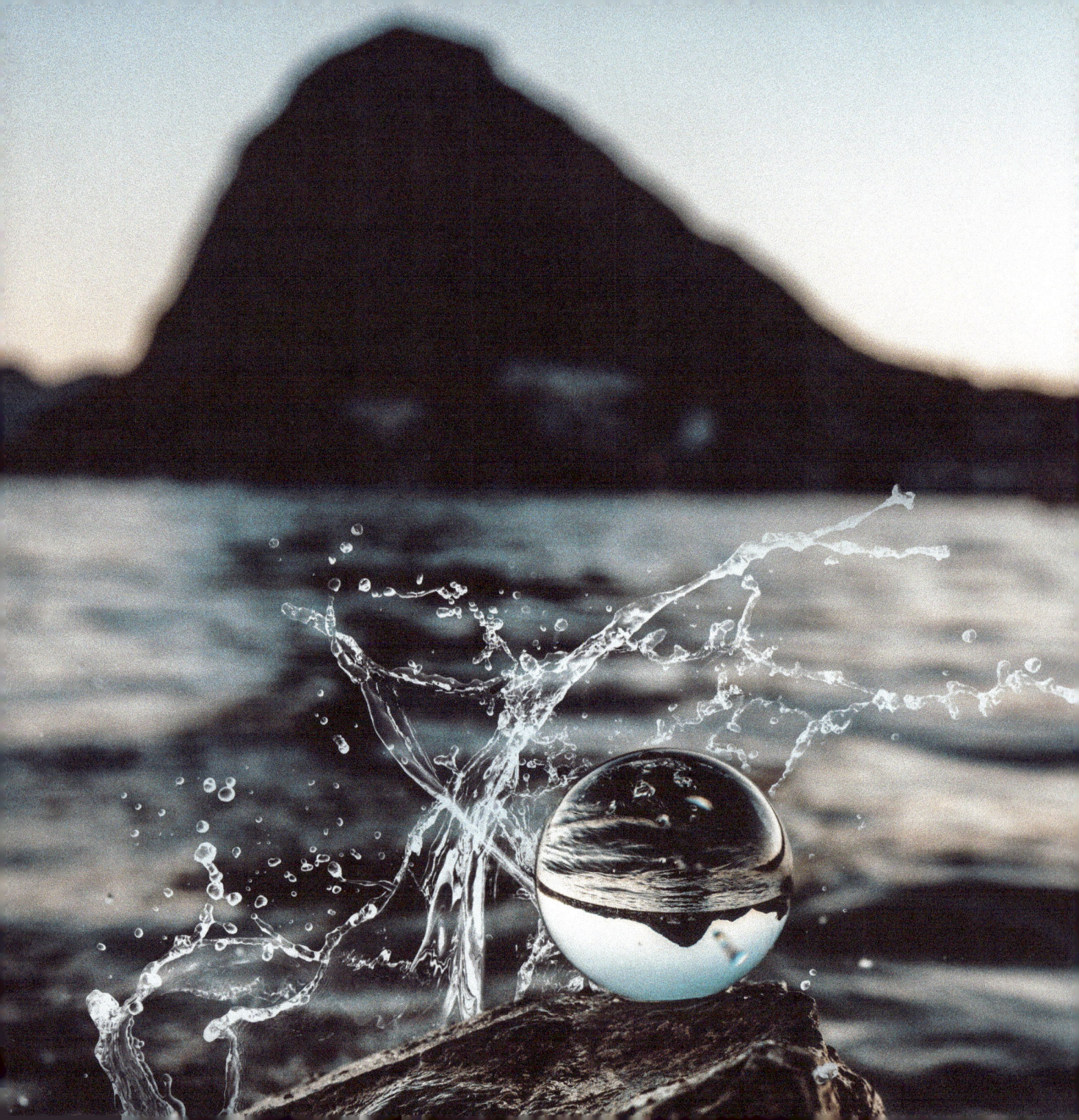

DRISHTI

The most common translation of *drishti* is "focused gaze." Although we can understand this more literally as the direction of our visual attention (and certainly, knowing where to physically look whilst within a Yoga posture can make all the difference), its contextual root is more so the mental gaze of concentration.

Let's break that down further:

What is concentration? What does it mean with respect to our physical organs and our known senses, to hold focus upon something? Quite like certain types of meditation (watching the breath or repeating a mantra), we take attention away from an unending number of other possible objects and place all of it upon one thing. Withdrawing the senses from any and all phenomena in our conscious awareness save for one—and layering all of those same efforts upon that one item.

Of course, holding a drishti in everyday life is the tiniest bit more complex than this breakdown would suggest, as the attention must always be divided, even if minimally so. When holding a Yoga pose, for example, some attention must be directed toward arranging the body into (and then holding) a certain physical shape. Another part of one's attention must be placed upon the breath.

Though it may not feel this way (especially as a new practitioner!), what remains of your well of energy over and above these elements is likely substantial, and a more robust practice means getting conscious and intentional about where to place that remaining attention.

In the context of mindfulness, we must ask ourselves how often our gaze is either backward or forward in time? Mindfulness meditation asks that we learn to notice our gaze and redirect it toward the only moment that exists, the only one that matters. On the mat as in life, where are we looking when our sense of balance is being challenged?

How aggressively are we looking?

Can we hold focus gently, but anchored at the same time?

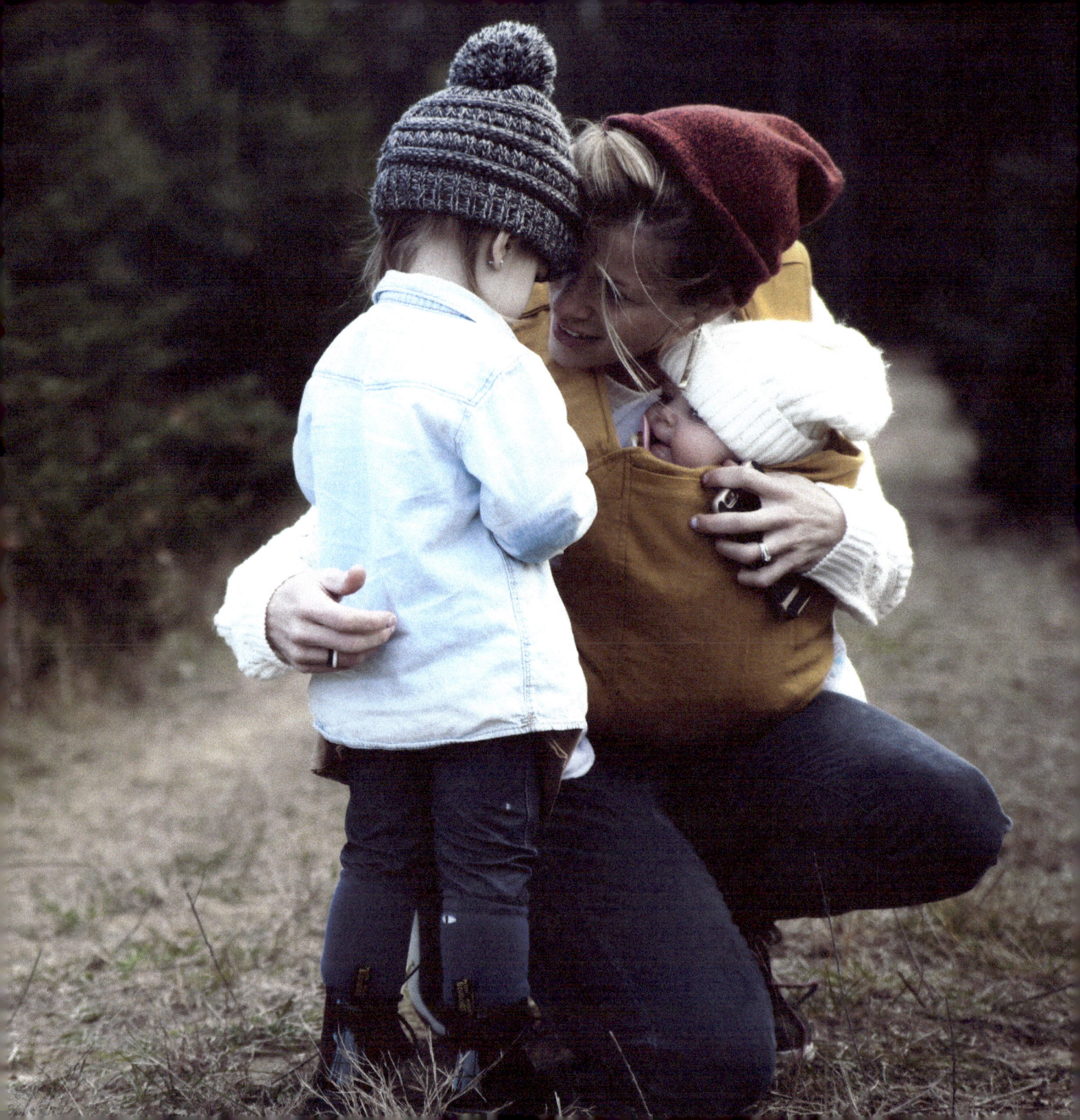

EQUANIMITY

"Equanimity, one of the most sublime emotions of Buddhist practice, is the ground for wisdom and freedom and the protector of compassion and love."
- Sayadaw U Pandita and Gil Fronsdal

In essence, it is observing without attachment nor emotional reaction, seeing with understanding. And at the same time, a balanced and calm state of mind in the midst of anything threatening this balance.

One exercise that helps us to train this skill is to draw two circles (on paper or in your mind), one larger, and one smaller within it.

Think about a situation that is currently stressful for you, and which is taking much of your energy. See if you can delineate which aspects of this situation are truly within your control (inner circle) and those which are not (outer circle).

Examples of things within your control: your response to something or someone, firm boundaries you could create, moving forward with a decision that is yours to make. Examples of things outside your control: someone else's attitudes/behaviors, decisions that are not yours to make, the weather... you get it.

For the smaller circle stuff, decide and act accordingly to better your circumstance in the ways you can. With anything you've placed in the outer circle, make a conscious choice to no longer engage with those things—not physically, mentally nor energetically.

When these items inevitably come up for you, see them, notice them, but as though watching a film. As though the witness only. They are not yours.

If we cannot control many or all of the forces external to us, can we maintain an inner composure through all of it? Throughout any situation, can we be present, mindful, lucid, level-headed, poised?

See if you can meditate or think on this today. The immensity of this concept and how you can cultivate a bit more of it in your life.

It will bring all of us inner peace, if we work at it in the small, consistent, everyday ways of mindfulness.

Find yourself calm, content, and composed in the middle of any storm.

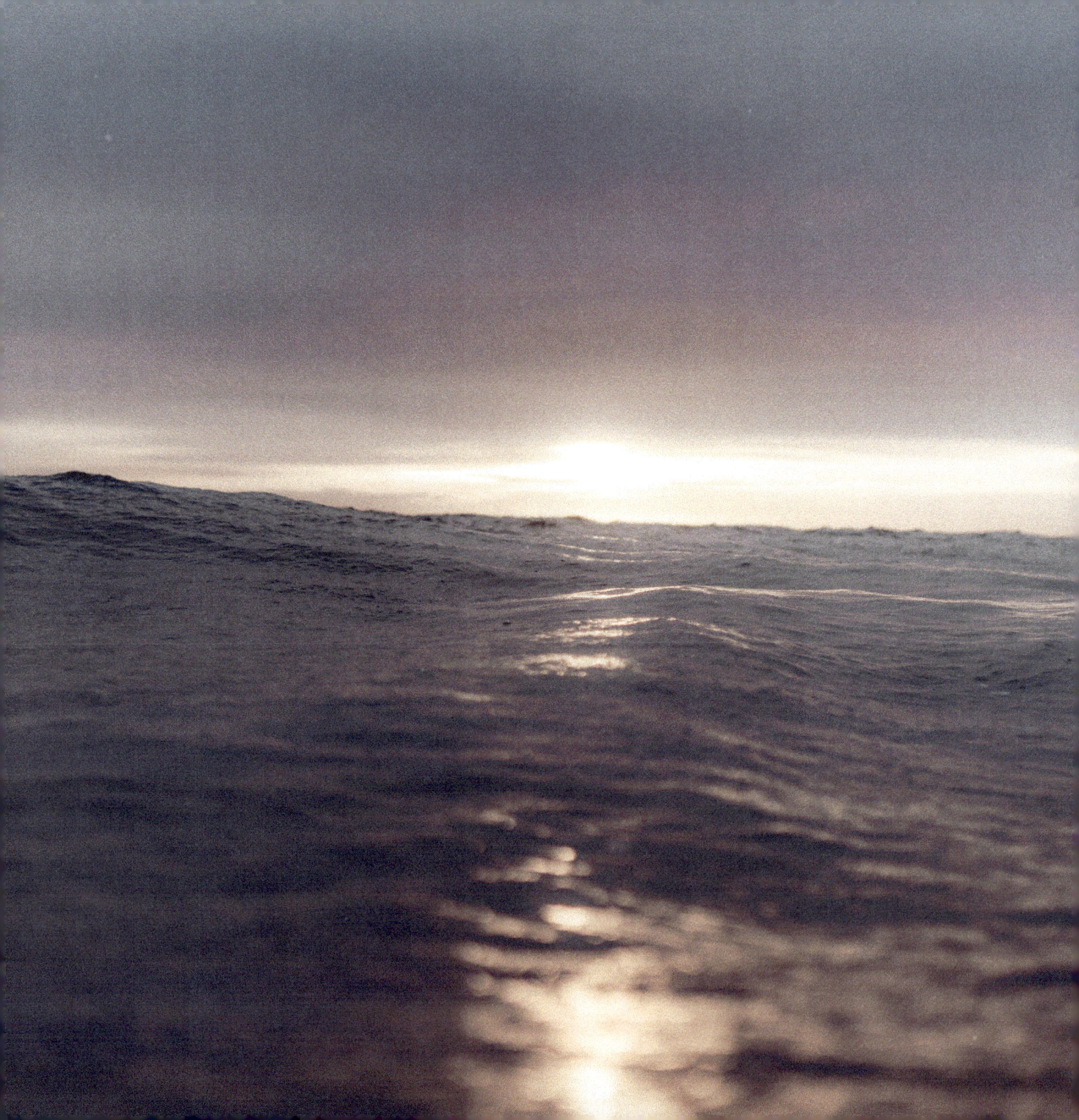

PRANA

If you've heard this term spoken it was likely in a yoga class, with reference to the breath or life force. Or maybe it was within the word *pranayama*—to restrain or draw out the breath as a means of controlling it (a technique, a practiced breath). This is a Sanskrit word with such depth of meaning it is difficult to pin it down while doing it justice. Still, having even the broadest sense of it works for most of us.

All the many forms of yoga hold prana and its awakening and control at their foundation.

In naturopathic medicine, we call this *the vis* (medicatrix naturae); the life force that resides in each and every one of us, responsible for our own health and healing. The word vitality is a good (however glib) approximation. Our treatments are meant to unblock stagnant energy, to revitalize a life force dimmed due to external or internal circumstance. Individuals are always the ones to heal themselves, via free-flowing vis or prana.

Prana allows us to have life, to act, to develop and to transform. It is both consciousness and creative power.

And if you take nothing else from this attempt at a definition, take this: Prana is not just the breath.

The breath is a graspable thing: *I get it, if I don't breathe,*

my cells die...it's a life force. And breathing practices are absolutely transformative.

It's *also*, importantly, that force which permeates mountains and the earth beneath our feet. The universe itself.

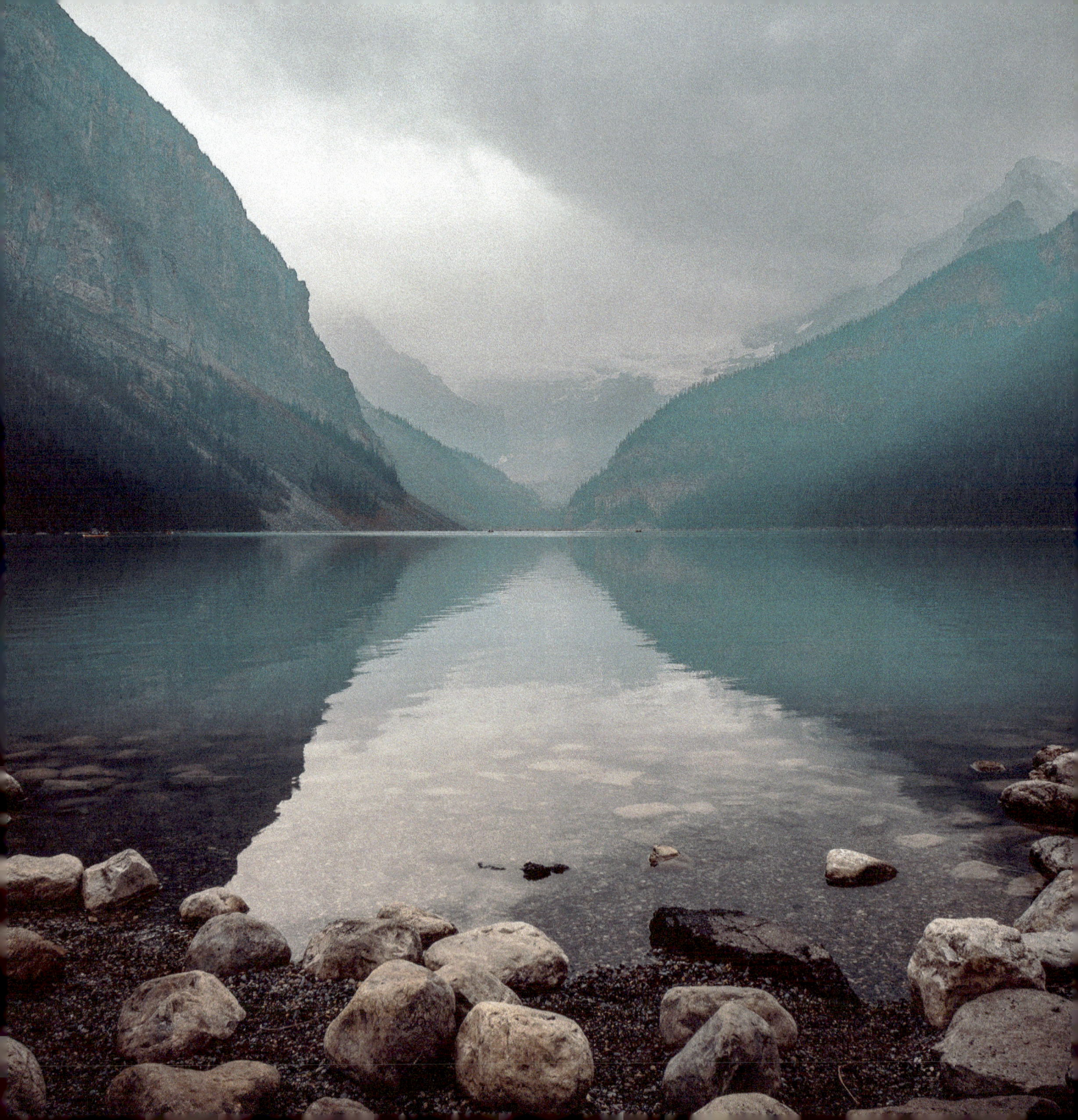

MINDFULNESS

It's hard to quite understand what we're talking about when we talk about mindfulness. The short history of this millennia-old practice goes as follows: Mindfulness is said to have arisen out of Vedic/Hindu, and later Buddhist, traditions (though some state it is also has roots in Islam, Christianity, and Judaism). Western mindfulness is most significantly influenced by Buddhist teachings, not the least of which is the idea of mindfulness being the first step on the path to Enlightenment. Of course, this is an oversimplification.

Mindfulness as a meditative practice is credited to Joseph Goldstein, Jack Kornfield and Sharon Salzberg who in 1975 created the Insight Meditation Society (IMS). Alongside the folks above, Jon Kabat-Zinn (whom I write about elsewhere in this text), is largely credited for bringing mindfulness to the West. He is the founder of the Centre for Mindfulness at the University of Massachusetts medical school and, in 1979, developed an eight-week stress reduction program to help chronically ill patients (what we now know as MBSR, or Mindfulness-Based Stress Reduction). He secularized the study as much as he possibly could, so as not to scare anyone away, focusing on the science.

Kabat-Zinn's definition is one of the most commonly quoted today: "Mindfulness is the awareness that arises from paying attention, on purpose, in the present moment and non-judgmentally".

He reminds us that a mindfulness practice is one which serves to build self-awareness and wisdom. The non-judgment piece is key—if we cannot take all of it lightly, if we cannot accept and love our wandering, often inattentive mind, it isn't mindfulness. Berating oneself for not being 'good' at the practice does not a wise mind build.

Thich Nhat Hanh (Zen Buddhist master), who was one of Kabat-Zinn's teachers, describes mindfulness more in terms of attention that is alive and awakened. He tells us that the conditions for our happiness are available to us "right here, right now". One need only recognize this and "stop running" to heal ourselves. We must be in that present moment, or rather, to continue to return to it, whether washing the dishes or observing a flower, with body and mind aware—completely alive.

Recognizing that our happiness is right here to be experienced, never a moment or a step away. Gratitude and acceptance play a significant role in this. More scientific attempts to understand and standardize mindfulness describe it as being about self-regulation and an openness and acceptance based on a curious mind.

Take your pick of ways to define it. But then get out of your head and practice.

Stop running.

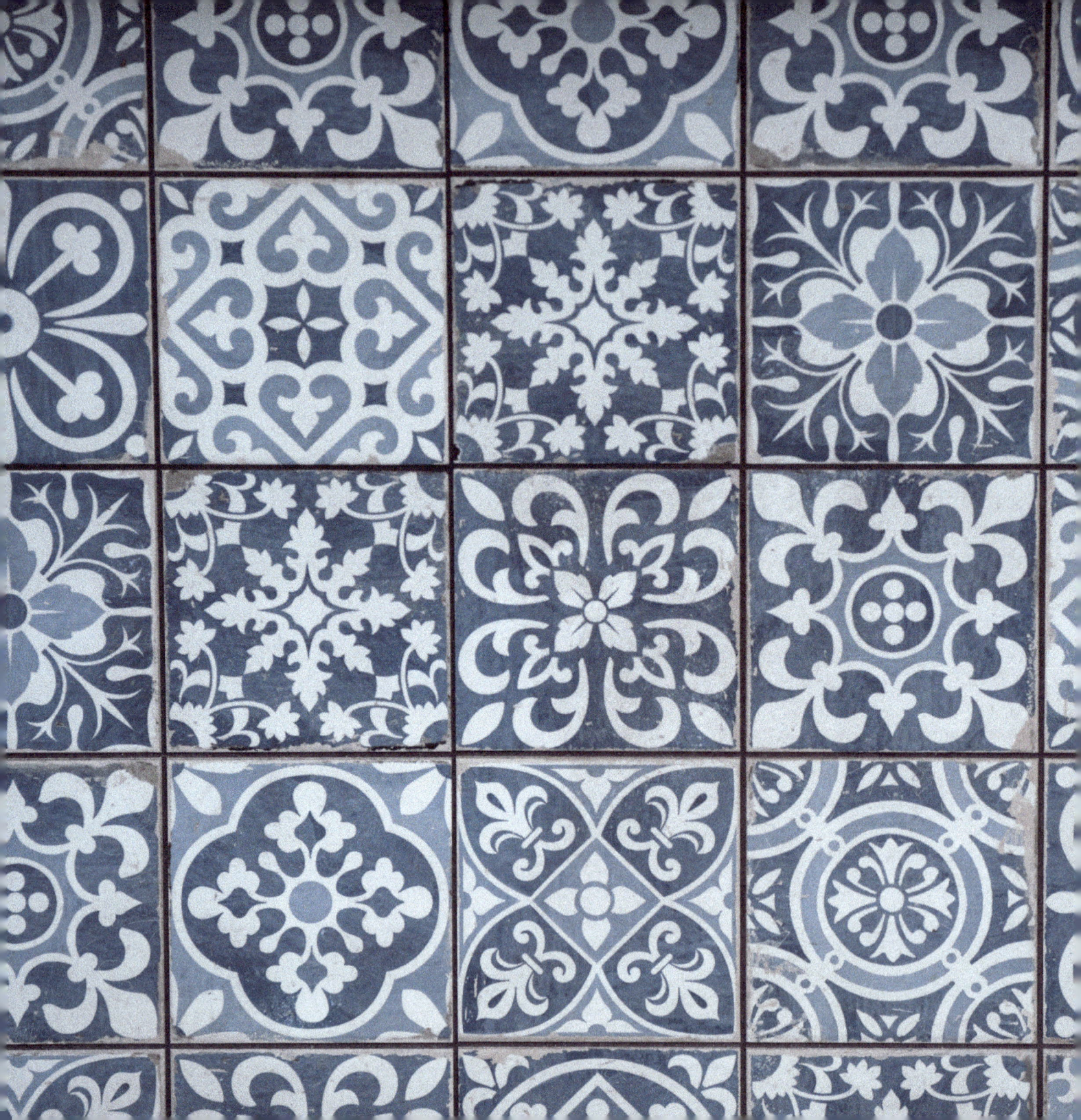

MANTRA

Pronounced 'MUNH-truh'. Also defined as a sacred utterance." If you're a yogi, you've likely been exposed to one or many mantras within the context of a class or meditation. These can be chanted, whispered, or merely spoken within, usually as a powerful meditative tool, to elicit a particular effect.

Some examples in Sanskrit:
- Sat Nam (I am Truth/Truth is my essence)
- Hari Om Tat Sat (The seen and unseen are both one)
- So Hum (I am That, all creation)
- Om / Aum: (The universal sound, the essence of consciousness)

Once again, I've significantly oversimplified by parsing these definitions down in this way—make no mistake, entire texts have been written attempting to approximate the true meaning of each. Please delve deeper if you're so called, books and the internet are your proverbial oysters.

If ancient languages aren't your thing, nowadays the word 'mantra' is used frequently outside of yogic/vedic circles to mean a phrase that is repeated to bring relief, peace and groundedness to the one uttering it. Something that keeps one steady and prevents an emotional or spiritual fall. As helpful as positive statements can be when repeated (I would term these affirmations rather than mantras), there is a reason we have kept alive the

Sanskrit syllables. The ancients have written about and passed down these phrases, to be spoken or chanted in their original form, emphasizing the sacred vibrations their sounds elicit. If you're looking for personal accounts of people having found incredible shifts via mantra practice, they abound. There has even been some research in cognition and neurology suggesting that mantra help our brain reduce distractions more effectively than other repetitive tasks.

In order to find one for you, speak to a teacher if you have one or take note if anything you read speaks to you when you speak it.

Beautiful, powerful, mood shifting sound.

Om Shanti.

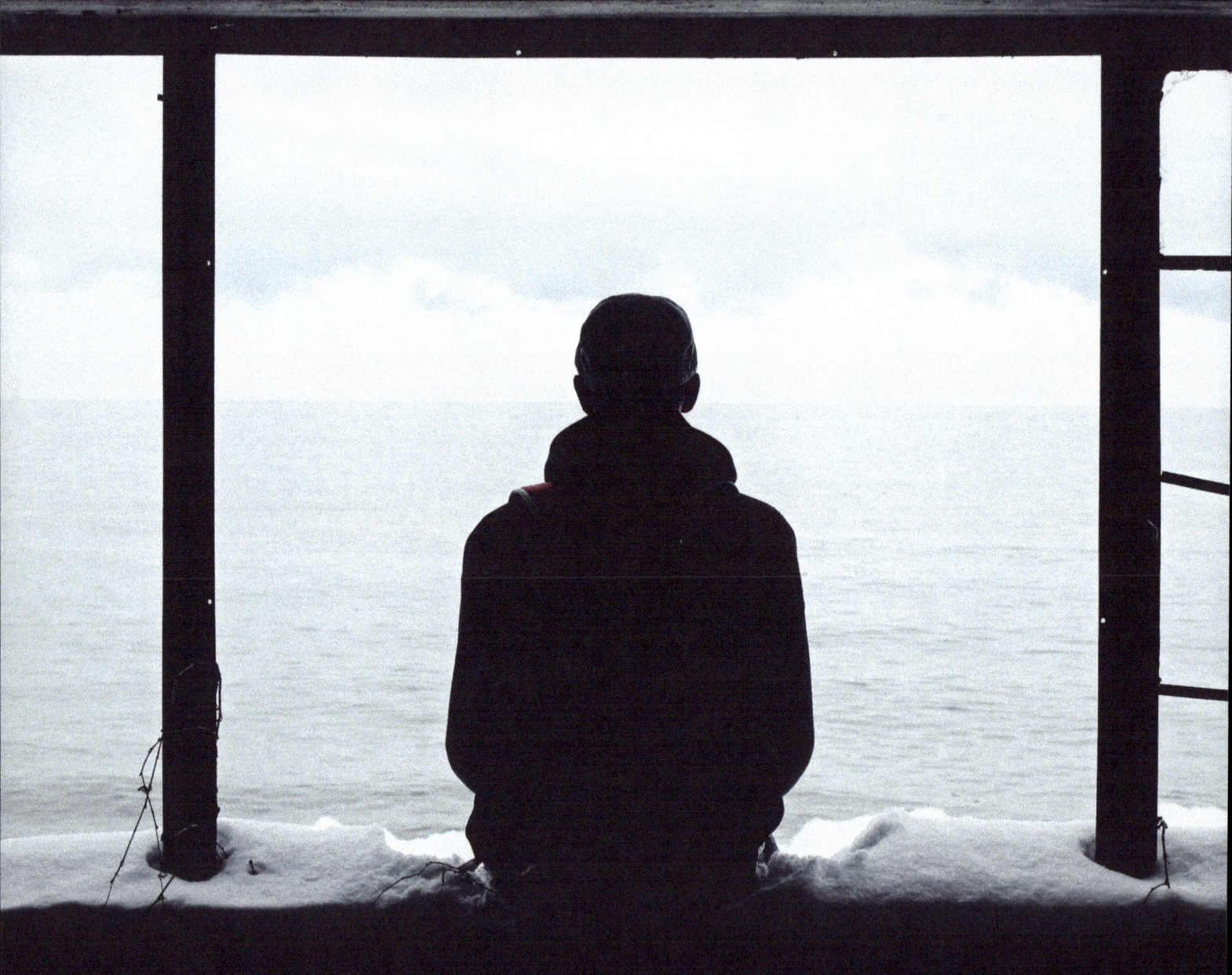

RUMINATION

Ever been caught in a pattern of thinking that made you feel horrible and yet seemed to trap you within it, however much you wanted out?

Rumination plays a very real and significant role in anxiety and depression. Negative thoughts and experiences find one another in brain and connect in neural networks. When any aspect of that network is triggered or recalled, the entire thing lights up like a string of Christmas tree lights. You may have heard that thoughts that wire together, fire together.

This is a well-known neuroscientific theory called Hebb's Rule or Hebbian Theory (after Donald Hebb in 1949). His cell assembly theory states that the more one neuron fires or excites its neighbor, the more efficient that connection becomes.

It makes sense that when we are feeling bad about ourselves in some way, previous times we experienced similar feelings then come to the fore, reinforcing the negative thought, and further strengthening all the things we'll revisit the next time such a thought is triggered. The double-edged sword of learning; it's a vicious and unfortunate cycle when we are prone to negative/anxious thinking. On the flip side, how wonderful for those who are naturally optimistic. If Hebb was right (and it appears he was), we can begin to appreciate how difficult it is to simply stop "going there." How seemingly impossible to just stop thinking the thoughts.

Psychology suggests that there is indeed hope on the other edge of that sword. Like anything else worth learning, it requires focused and repeated effort in the other direction: Purposeful remembering of positive moods, thoughts, memories, and self-image. Actively recalling when things went well for you, despite initial fear, anxiety, or trepidation. Positive rememberings from friends and family and happy sensorial memories (music, tastes, smells, physical sensations from joyful times) are potent tools.

Of course, mindfulness meditation is one of the most powerful and effective practices to stop rumination and instead be willful about where we place our attention, when, and for how long. To the monkey mind that thinks it's got us controlled, it's basically kryptonite.

Arm yourself.

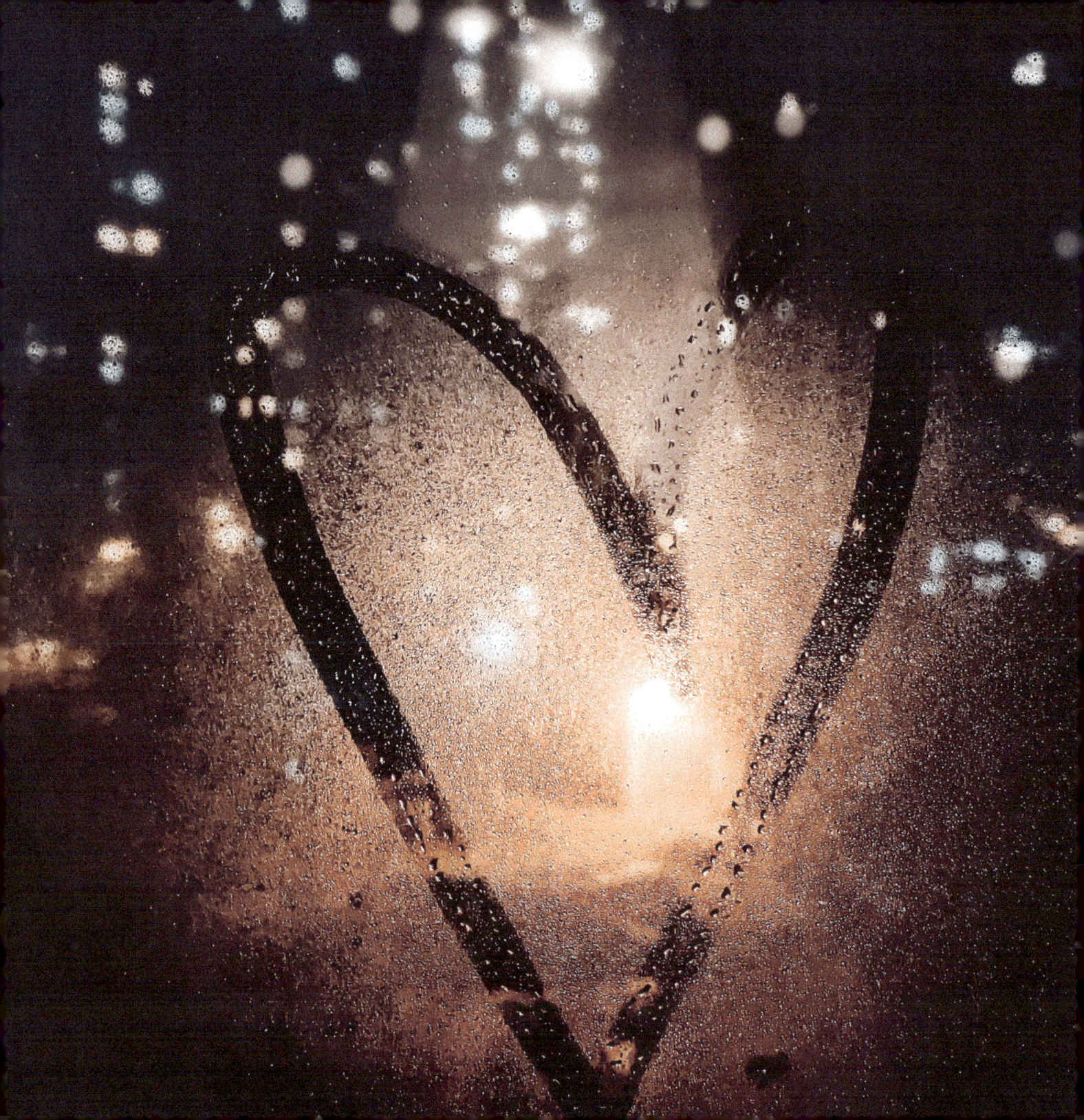

AHIMSA

If I could hold onto one word as a guide, for the remainder of my life, it would be this. Such rich meaning in one six-letter word.

Somewhere between 200 and 500 BCE, the Indian sage, Patanjali, brought us the yoga sutras—a compilation of the traditional understandings of yoga in all its forms (philosophy, practice). One section discusses the eight limbs of yoga. Two such limbs are the Yamas (abstinences) and Niyamas (observances). Essentially, these are guidelines to follow if one is on the path to liberation/fulfillment.

I like to think of Yamas as DO NOTs and Niyamas as DOs. Ahisma, the first of the Yamas, tells us to avoid violence and harm. Vitally, this refers to others as well as to ourselves. It is meant to describe all forms of violence or harm including hurtful words and thoughts, as these can be equally, if not more, injurious than actions.

The practice of Ahimsa really underscores every aspect of how we live and how we choose to be. What negative thoughts might we be having about ourselves or others, when in pursuit of something "good"? The damage done may outweigh any kind intention. This really calls us to look at the totality of our energetic inputs and outputs, the butterfly effects, near and far, upon ourselves and others. What are the peripheral (though not lesser) effects of that action/phrase/habit/self-talk? Importantly, Ahimsa does *not* mean allowing and accepting just

anything along the path of non-harming. It underscores acting intentionally and lovingly with eyes open—holding us responsible for minimizing harm in both directions.

Preserving and caring equally for ourselves and others is the essence of this sacred practice.

As with all sound guidance, the dos and don'ts aren't always so clear. Context matters. We are tasked with this invaluable responsibility and have to make our own choices from our own discerning, all-loving hearts.

Ahimsa is, to me, the greatest possible guiding principle.

So, we practice.

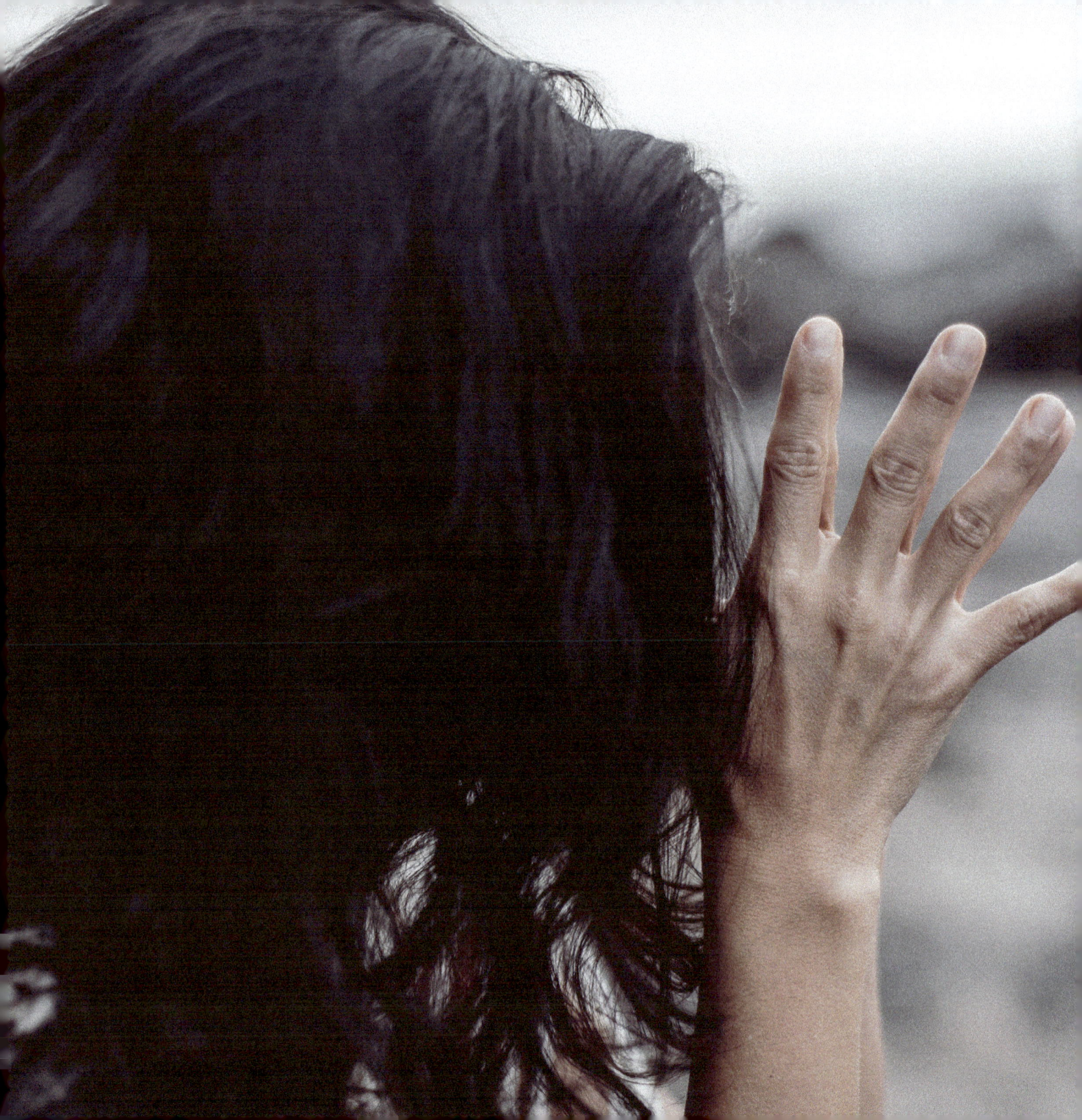

NAMASTE

Likely the most commonly used, abused, and mis-used Sanskrit word in the West. Commonly used with kind intention at the end of yoga classes in a slight bow to the teacher. Anyone on social media or the internet at all (!) can attest to seeing at least one hilarious meme mocking this otherwise beautiful acknowledgment.

So, what are we saying when we reverently say *namaste*? You may have read it summarized as "the light in me recognizes and honors the light in you," or simply, "my soul honors your soul." Usually, this is a gesture directed to a teacher, or to a fellow student. When used with genuine feeling and ego forfeited, it can create a strong union between the two parties. It can be equally used toward oneself, in meditation, to find deeper introspection.

We place the palms of the hands together, either at the heart chakra (physical area of the centre of the chest, energetic area of joy, compassion, and unconditional love) or at the third eye (between the eyebrows, the space of intuition and inner knowing). Usually, the eyes are closed and there is a gentle bow of the head as well.

In India and other parts of Asia, children learn early on to greet their elders with namaste and/or with the symbolic hand gesture. To family, to neighbors, to essentially everyone. It is a common, heartfelt "hello".

In a yoga class, when the teacher initiates the namaste gesture to their students, they are acknowledging their own past teachers while at the same time opening the line of spiritual communication with their present students. The students respond in kind. In this exchange, there is a transfer of respect, gratitude, and Truth.

The best way I've heard this described is ubiquitous as it is profound: *I honor the place in you where the entire universe resides. I honor the light, love, truth, beauty, and peace within you because it's also within me. In sharing these things, we are united, we are the same, we are one.*

We are one.

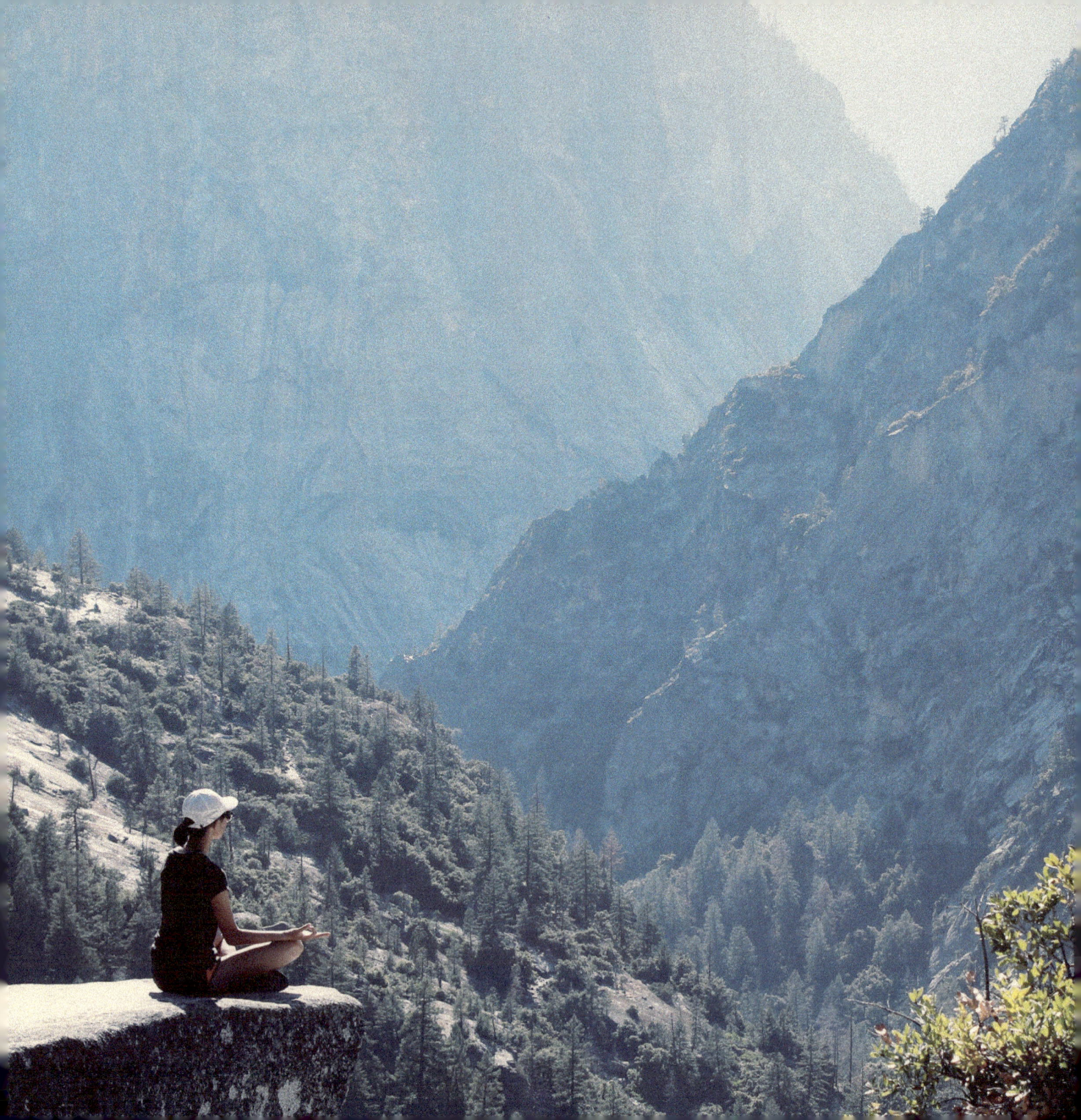

VIPASSANA

Buddhism describes two major categories of meditation. In the Pali language, these are *Samatha* (translates as concentration/tranquility) and *Vipassana* (translates as insight/clarity), the latter being the oldest form of Buddhist meditation known. Though most traditional meditation practices fall under one of these two umbrellas, with all of the various influences, you may have experienced styles that contained aspects of either or both.

In Samatha, or concentration practice, we learn to focus all attention on a *singular* object/word/image/breath etc. and in excluding all other thoughts, a beautiful calm comes over the meditator whilst sitting. This type of practice is the perfect training ground for becoming more task-focused in everyday life; learning the skill of attending to the thing you want to attend to and disregarding all the others. Being less scattered. With this practice, we can achieve (impermanent) moments of focus where the usually busy mind quiets and thoughts outside of our desired attention aren't actually arising.

In Vipassana, the student is called to an awakening that is quite distinct. Here, we are waking to the nature of consciousness and one's ability to see everything within it for what it truly is, regardless of how many ubiquitous inputs are vying for our attention. The more complete terminology is Vipassana Bhavana. *Vipassana*—to see straight through and into and with full clarity, and *Bhavana*—to cultivate the mind. It is essentially the study of

cultivating a state of mindfulness, or simply, a mindfulness-*based* meditation practice. Elements of concentration meditation are useful especially in the beginning stages of this study, so attending to the breath is often an early component. Take note, despite its Buddhist roots, Vipassana can be (and is often) taught and practiced in a wholly secular way.

Ever known a friend or colleague who told you they were going off-grid for ten days on a silent retreat? Where not only was speaking mostly forbidden but writing or reading of any kind as well? Did you think they were crazy? Vipassana retreats are well known and very popular in meditator circles.

For Buddhist practitioners, years and years of dedicated practice are said to lead to the religion's chief goal: liberation, freedom from suffering. Steadily, little by little, one's understanding concerning what truly lies within and beyond us—underneath the illusory version of truth we have always believed—grows. It starts simply enough, with an attention on the breath. Again, you need not be a Buddhist to engage in it, nor be an experienced meditator. You need to have a pulse and carry breath. The promise of true, enlightened contentment. The promise of becoming fully awake to what really is.

Sit with that.

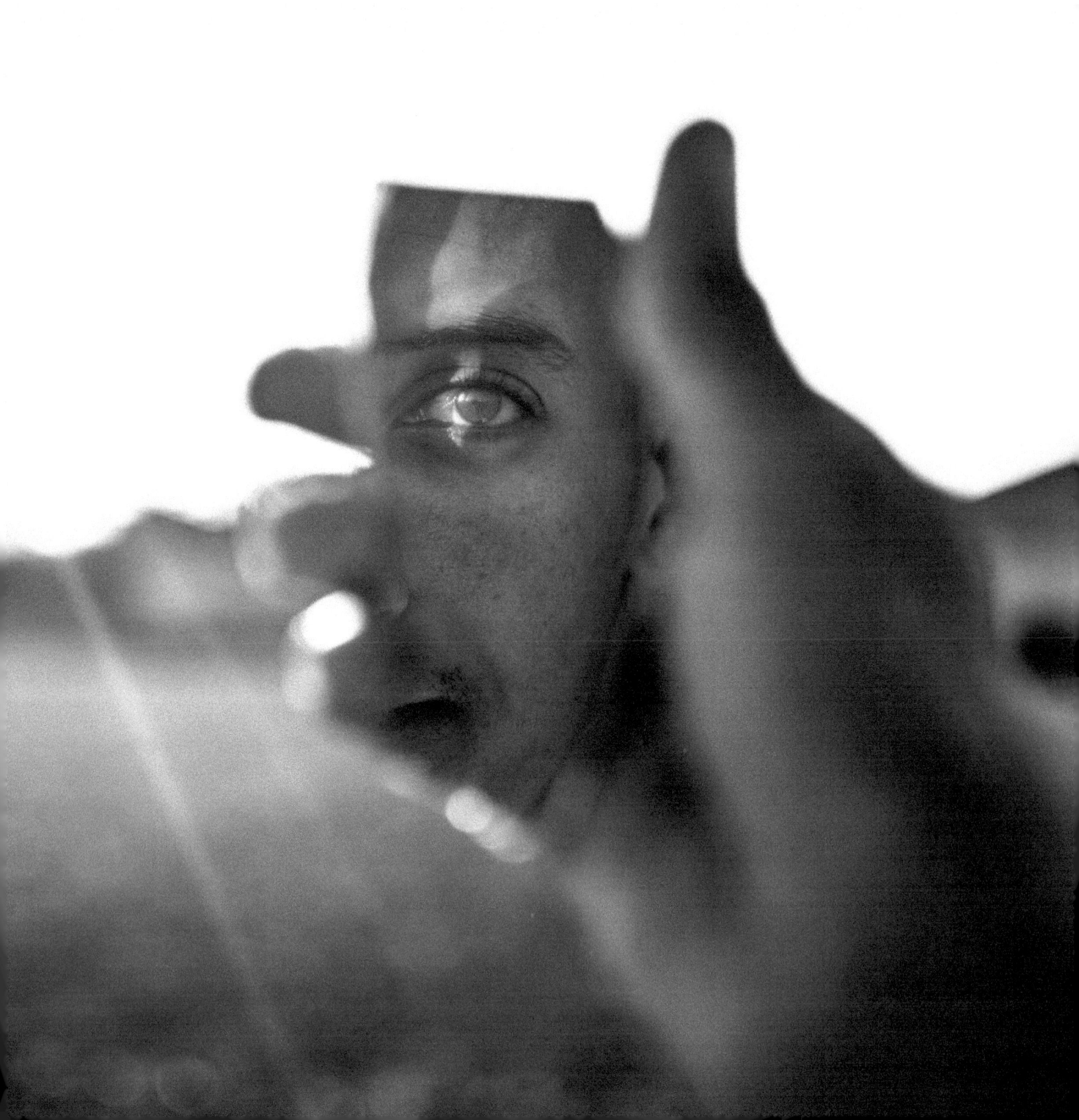

EGO

Like most complex and layered concepts, this term gets tossed around the common vernacular in so many ways it's difficult to pin down its true meaning. Here are some of the predominant views:

The ego is not inherently bad. It is all things "I," "me," "my," and "mine". It's what some might deem *Identity*, the collective decisions, thoughts, opinions, actions, words, emotions, and experiences that make up one's *Self*. Most of us perceive that each identity is precisely all those things combined. It rings accurate that I am indeed the collection of all those things, and that these, when packaged together, are what separate me from everybody else. That it is specifically the contrast between this collection and that collection which defines how I am I, and how I am *not them*. Usually, this definition takes as given that there is a thinker, an experiencer, a permanent, unitary *je-ne-sais-quoi*, housed somewhere in the mind, which is driving the bus. Here, the ego is on the edge of consciousness, observing all things outside and separate from itself. There is I, and there is the rest.

A viewpoint found in some Yogic/Hindu/Buddhist traditions is that the ego is simply an earthly suit with moving parts which conceals the true self—pure consciousness. It is seen as the necessary vehicle for the stretch of highway between where we are and self-actualization: the pure bliss that is to come when we fully wake to the profound Truth within.

Within the 'personal contracts' that we must fulfill on the path of yoga, *Svadhyaya* (or, self-inquiry) is one. To reach liberation, one must actively study the ego until the 'I' is revealed. And at the precise moment it is revealed, it dissolves—the ego is transcended.

Non-dualists go even further. Their perspective is that there is, in fact, no ego nor self to speak of. That there is no one on the edge, observing all the phenomena within consciousness. Instead, that every single thought, emotion, and sensory input each of us may experience *is us*.

For non-dualists, the ego is an illusion. We are not experiencing consciousness, rather, we are the exact same as consciousness. There is no separation.

What's in an ego?

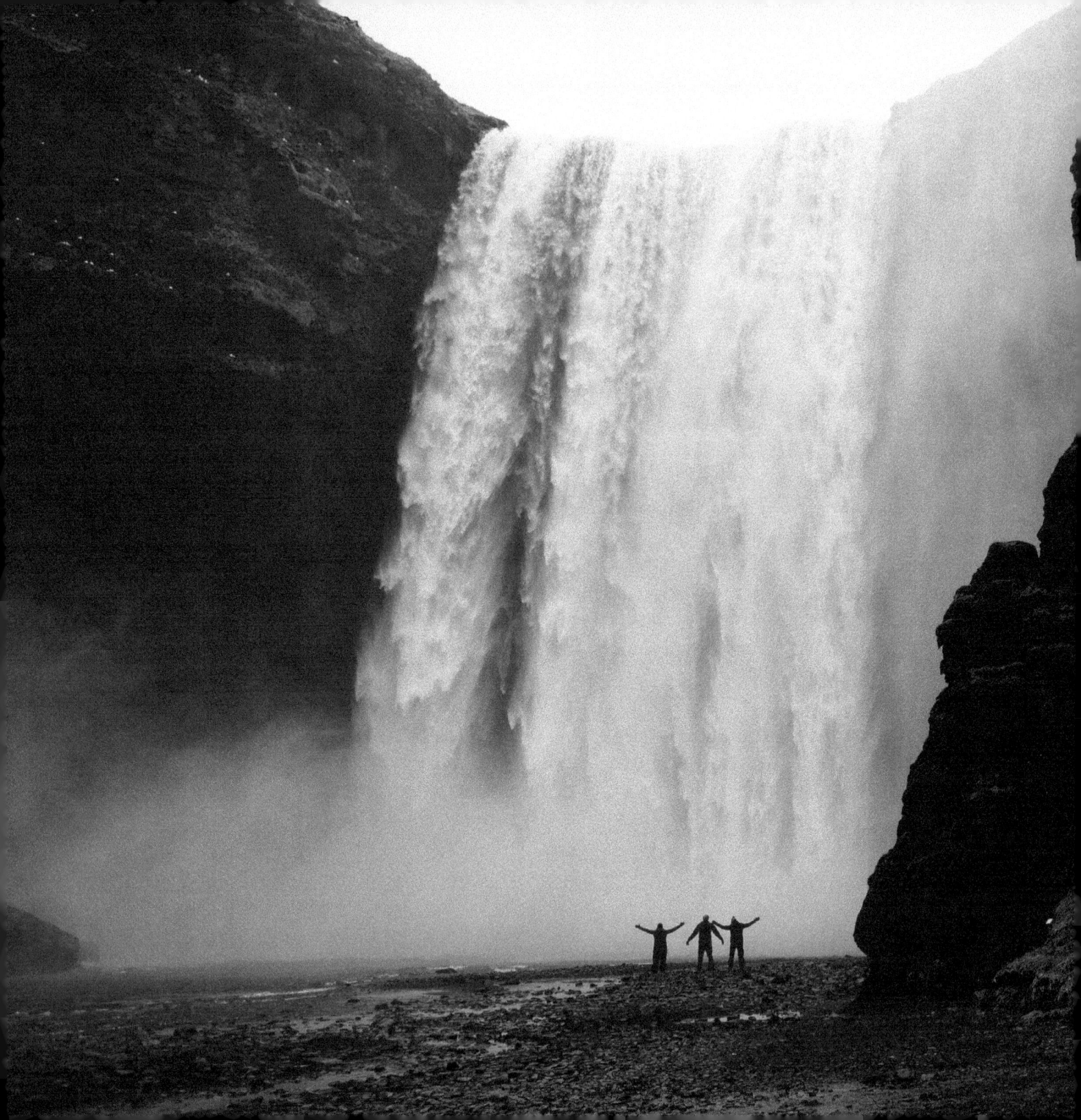

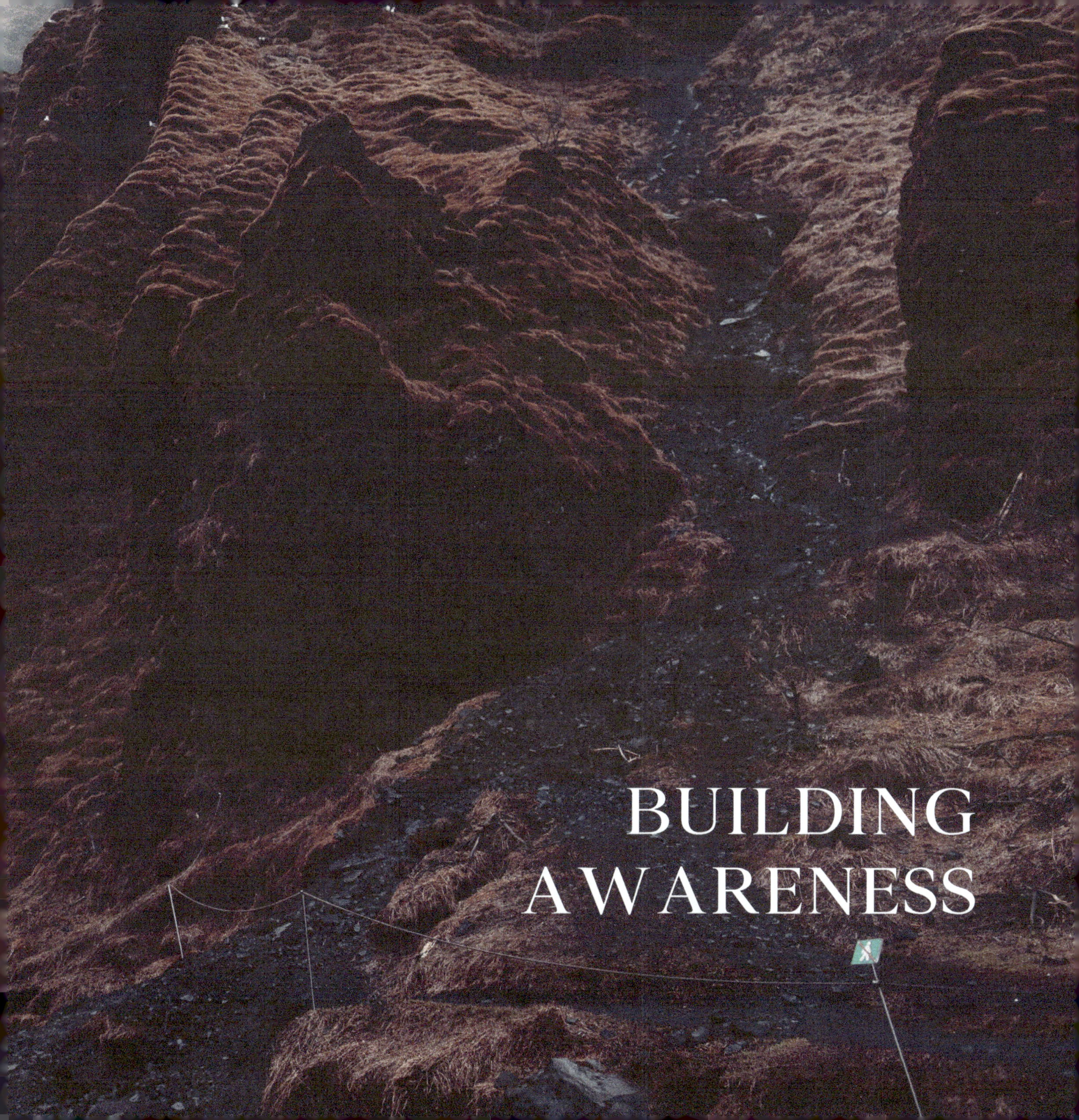

BUILDING
AWARENESS

AWARENESS

Are you fully awake?

I've found that one of the biggest barriers to my patients feeling better (i.e. the most limiting obstacle to cure) is a partial or complete lack of self-awareness. Letting go of the concept of an illusory self [see "Ego" in the Language section], self-awareness, the way I see it, is being cognizant of what is happening in one's mind, body, and spirit, and sensing when one or more aspects have shifted. In healthcare, it's the difference between you informing your doctor that something is off, and having your doctor inform you.

So many of us are simply not aware of the nuances of our physical, mental, and emotional selves. At times, the connection may be completely lacking; say, being the last one to notice your recent aggression, or being wholly unaware of shifts in energy throughout the day or week. Other times, there is a modicum of self-awareness but there is missing data. You may recognize, for example, that you are often irritable, but not fully conscious of your triggers. You may feel physical discomfort or pain and yet be unable to connect the aspect of your diet or environment that provoked it.

As with everything, the skill of thorough self-awareness is born of and strengthened by practice. We practice by choosing to draw attention toward something, by tapping in, by intentional noticing. It requires getting curious about all the things we are noticing on a deeper level. Like exploring different senses that you will indeed have access to only if you get interested and listen very closely.

We will never be able to heal ourselves if we do not get to know ourselves.

The prompts in this section will be dedicated to helping you in this very pursuit. Use them while going about the things you find yourself going about, day to day. Rather than a sitting practice, this is about getting conscious within the context of your waking, walking, everyday life.

For those who feel they have no spare moment to sit and meditate, know that a daily attention practice is another, quite effective, way of cultivating mindfulness. Rather than asking us to judge or change our actions or attitudes, the only rule is that we bring a different quality of attention to a specific aspect of our experience.

Whether you practice it for a few minutes at a time, for an entire day or week... know that each time you bring your mind to it, you strengthen the muscle further.

By getting truly curious, we awake.

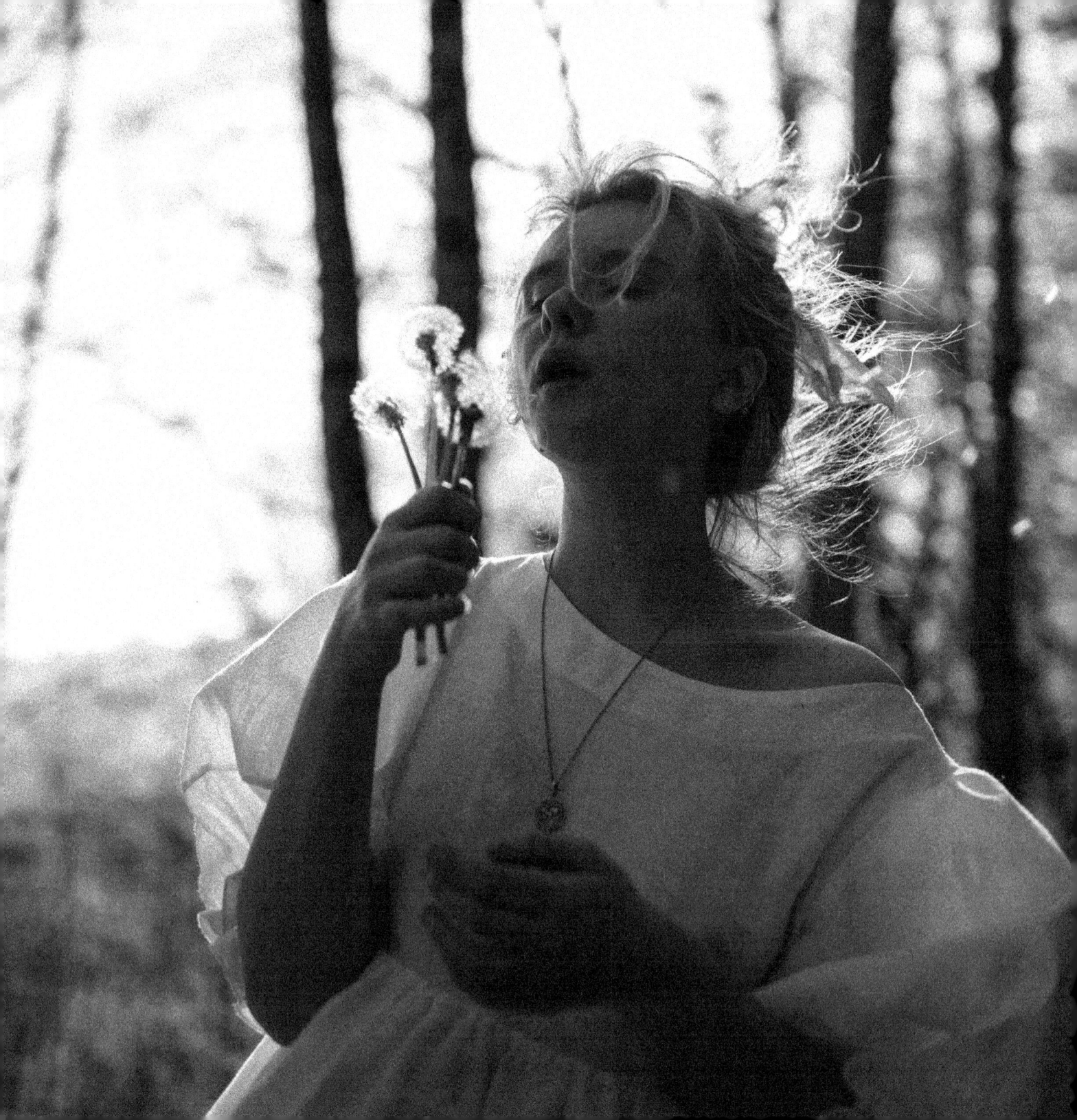

BREATH

Wake up to your breath.

This is foundational.

The breath is a barometer for most aspects of our human systems—whether our nervous system, our mood, or our sense of physical and emotional ease or discomfort.

Pause for a moment to pay attention to your inhale, exhale, the pauses before, between and after. Is it slow or fast, regular, or choppy, audible, or quiet? Does it arise from your shoulders, your belly, or elsewhere?

How does it reflect your current mental-emotional state? Your physical one?

Just notice. No need to change what you notice in any way.

Later on, repeat the exercise and note if anything has changed. Continue in this way as many times as you can remember before the day is through.

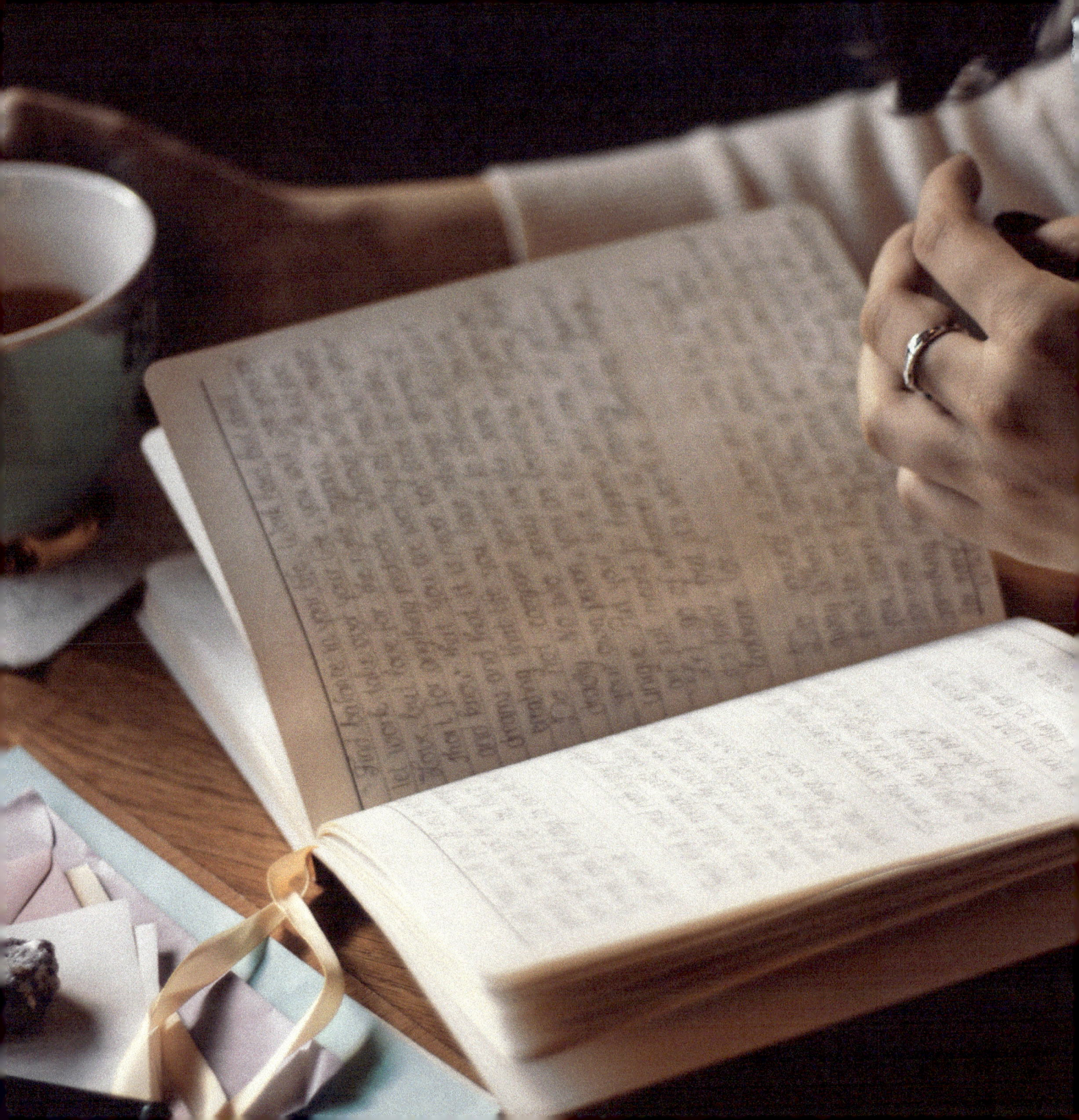

WORDS

Wake up to the words you are using to express yourself.

Notice the language you are using to speak to those around you.

Are the words precise? Kind? Honest? Accurate? Do they leave too much in or too much out regarding the message you would like to share? Are they conveying exactly what you intend?

Pay attention to whether you are making moment-to-moment choices when speaking, or on automatic pilot using a long-established language pattern.

When asked a question, are you employing standard phrases to fill the gap, or are you clearly communicating a genuine response?

Do you use certain words with some people and not with others?

Of course, words are just one aspect to expression. But for today, pay attention to this only.

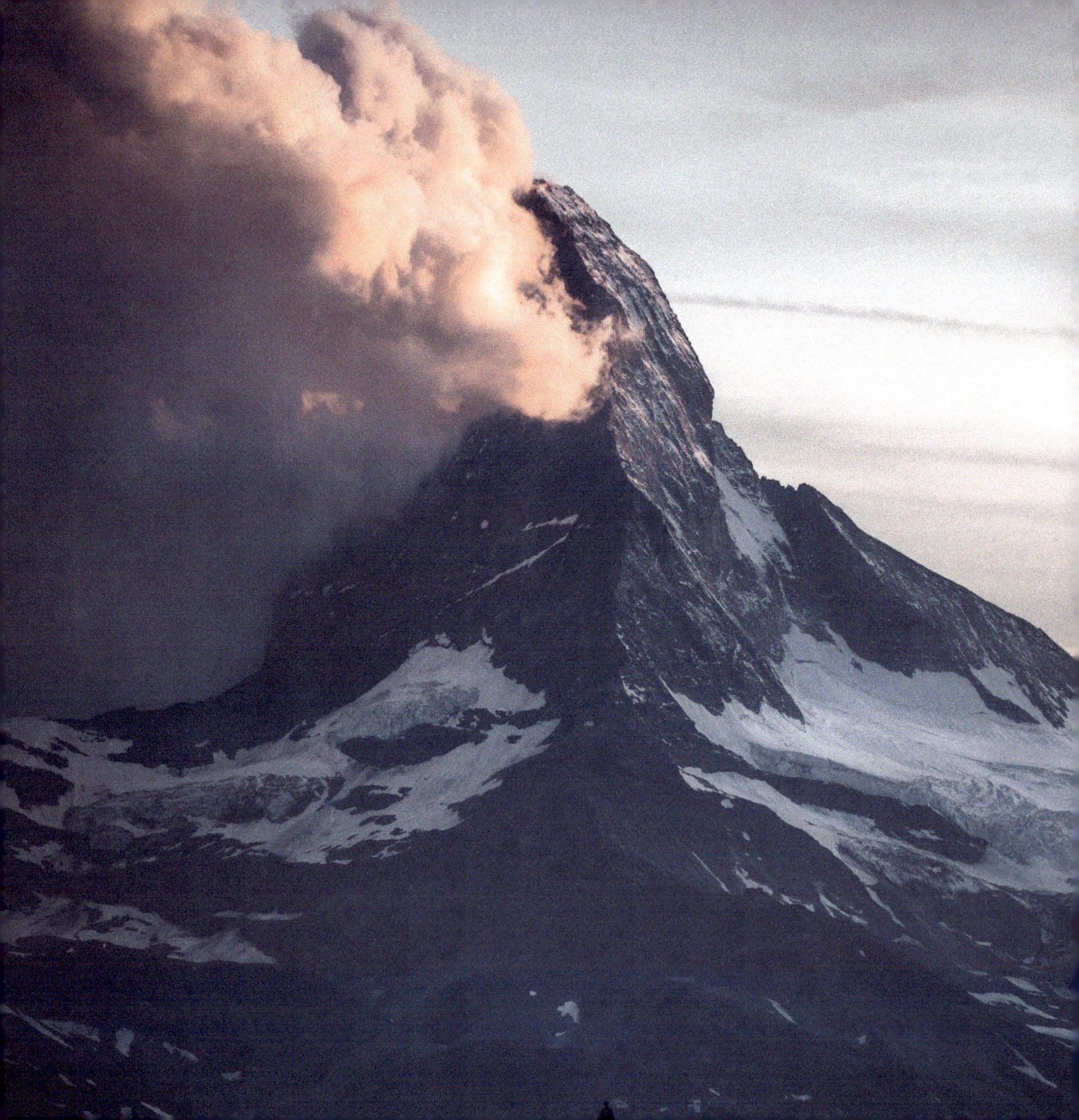

MOOD

Notice your mood at various points throughout the day. It will fluctuate.

Ask:
- Why did I wake up already in mood x or y?
Can you link it to a yesterday event? A rabbit-hole line of thinking you humanly followed but which really didn't help or feed you?

Then ask:
- Do I want to keep that going or do I want to choose anew?
Who and how do you want to show up today? Every single minute is a new moment to choose again, to break the rut. A new opportunity to disrupt the automatic copy-and-pasting of what came before and instead see the open space that lies before you.

And then, decide.

Feel powerful and responsible and totally in control as you choose what you want to put out into the world in that moment.

What mood would you like to share and have cross over onto your colleague, friend, partner, child, parent, pet? And so importantly, what do we want to reinforce to *our-selves?*

Because we are not islands.

And how we feel and what we choose to hold onto is always, inevitably, shared.

In your difficult moment, do you want your cup of sadness/pain/confusion/overwhelm/fear to spill over onto your circle of people and then, cruelly, receive it back again?

Or is what you need most right now to receive the opposite state of mind in return?

We create our emotional environments.

Stop unkindly waiting for kindness to shower you. Choose your environment right now.

Then do it again. And then again.

47

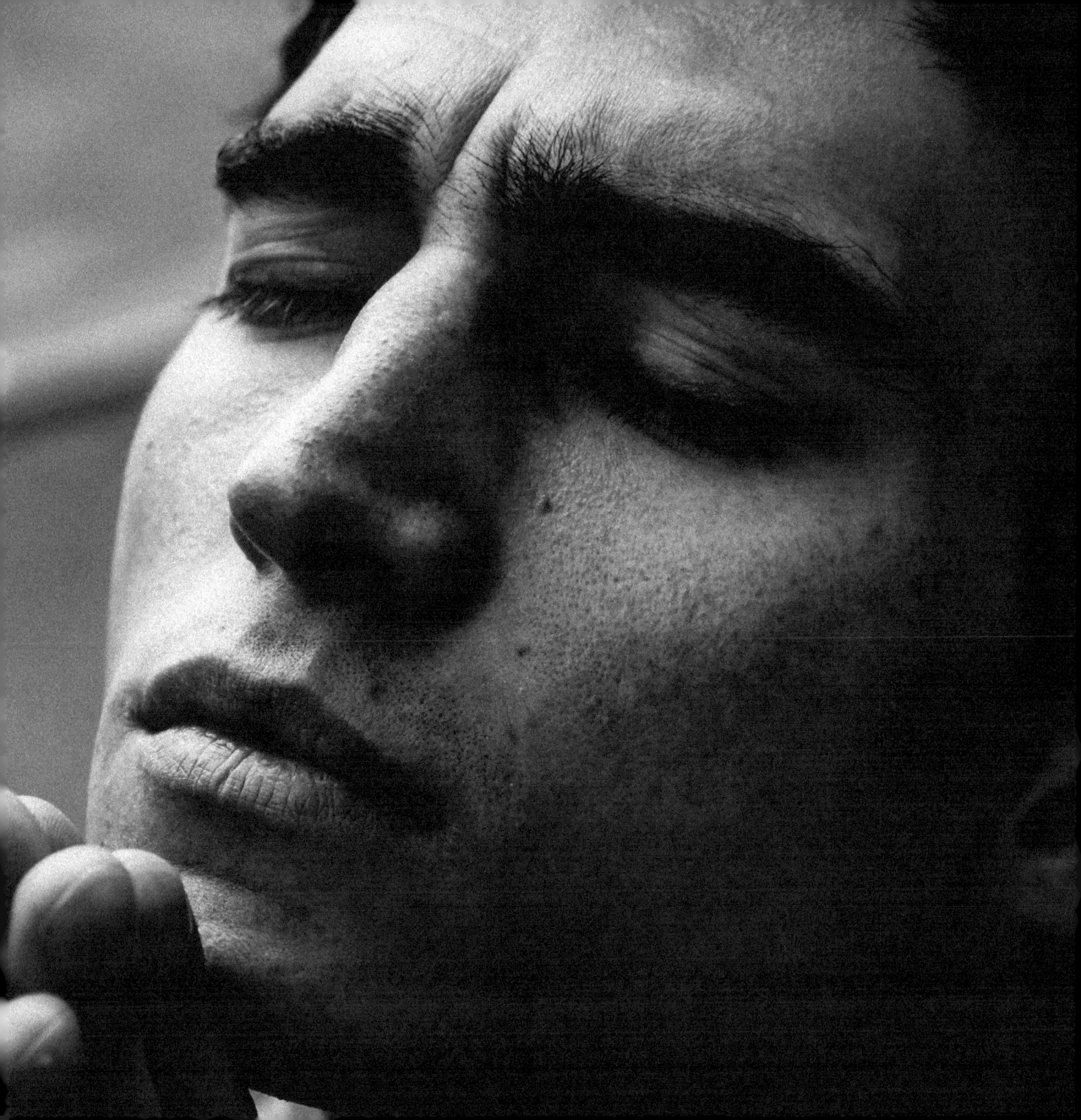

TENSION

Wake up to the holding patterns in your body.

In what ways do you notice you tense up, subconsciously, when involved in the distractions of work or life stress?

Perhaps, even, in neutral daily tasks?

Common patterns:
- shoulders hunched (forward and up towards ears)
- chin forward
- teeth / jaw clenched
- belly tight
- holding breath
- eyebrows furrowed / tense
- biting (inside lip / cheek, nails)
- repetitive micro movements (skin picking, touching face, foot tapping)

Notice whatever way your body is used to holding tension. See if every time you bring awareness to it you can consciously let that tension go. Take a deep breath into that place. Set yourself reminders to do this a few times today. You may notice that the tension doesn't just automatically melt away by virtue of a few moments of recognition. Reversing these holding patterns takes continued awareness and repeated, conscious un-tensing.

How much of our anxiety, overwhelm, chronic pain, poor posture, poor sleep, etc. could be reversed with this simple, repeated awareness?

The reason why most people won't follow this advice is because they still believe that their healing lies in a pill or a procedure or something 'big', singular, and external.

Hear this now: it's in the small, consistent, and continual. The real healing lies within you.

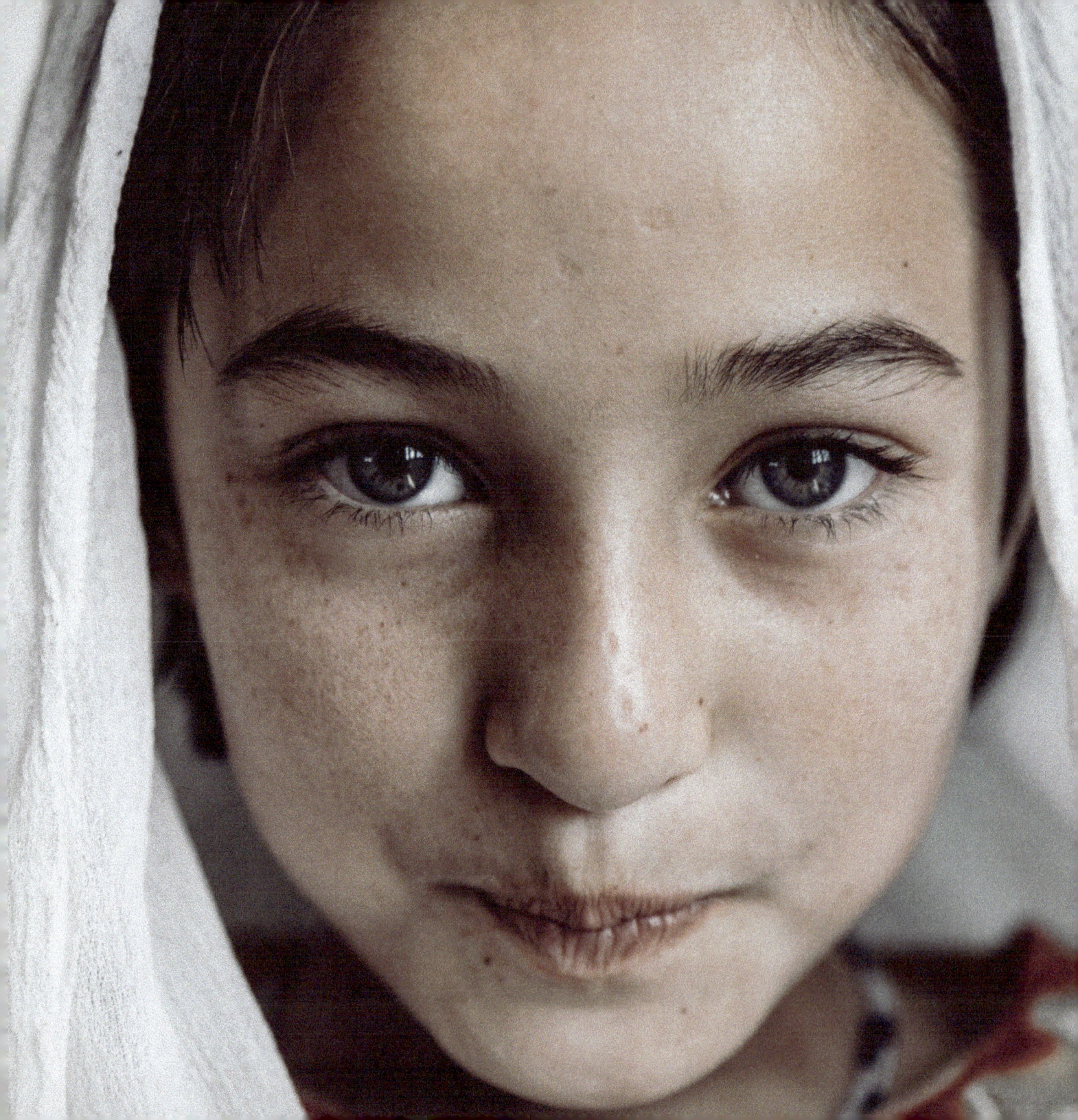

EXPRESSION

Wake up to what the look on your face is really saying, behind what you may be speaking.

Facial expression. Such a great proportion of what we communicate to the world and of the messages we receive from others is below conscious awareness.

Have you ever heard of micro-expressions? These are lightning fast (under half a second) automatic facial responses stemming from the brain's amygdala which result from trying to conceal a true emotion—conveying what are deemed the "seven universal emotions": fear, anger, disgust, contempt, sadness, happiness, and surprise.

Although scientists in this field say these are undetectable to the naked eye (using slow motion cameras to capture them accurately), I'd argue that, when emotionally connected to someone, there is a subconscious feeling of deeper knowing that something is off, something doesn't feel honest, when any true emotion is concealed.

It's notable, too, that our continual, changing display of macro-expressions are usually a suffficient way to reveal how we're really feeling inside. Often despite ourselves.

Today, notice how you hold the aspects of your face. Your eyes, your lips, your cheeks, chin, nose, and brow.

Become aware of the emotions expressed in the looks you display, especially when engaged in conversation.

It can be useful to ask a loved one what your facial expression is saying from their perspective to gain insight. If you are truly open to learning about yourself, this exercise can be a profound eye-opener and may help soften interactions that were once challenging.

Wake up to your expression:
What are you saying to the world?
Shouldn't you know?

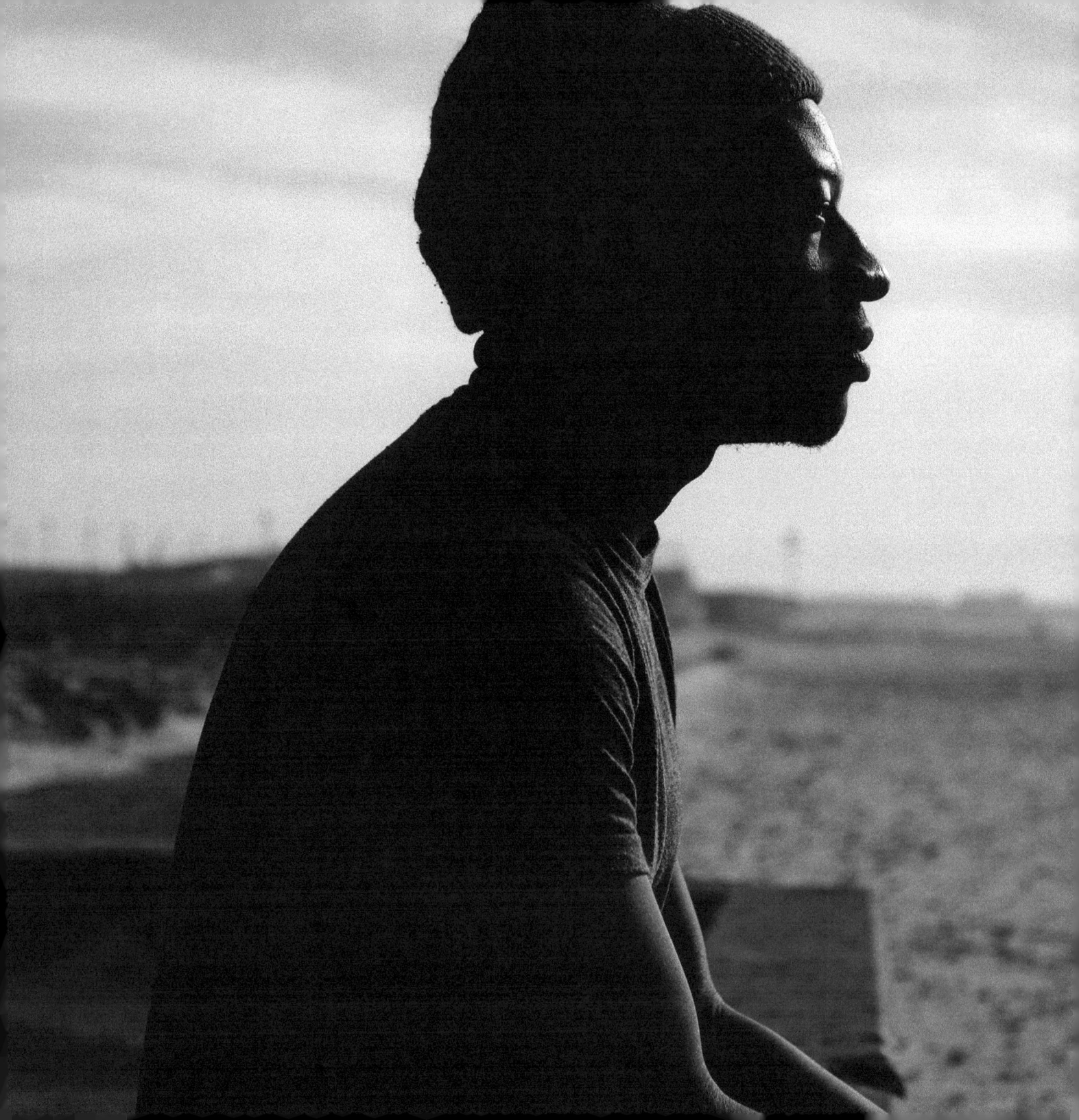

THOUGHTS

Wake up to your thoughts. You know, those little love-them or hate-them gems swimming around in your head.

Are they the half-full type, or half-empty?
Are they even accurate?

Let's remember that we are always decoding information from the world, contextually. That is, as it occurs and relates to our circumstance and current state of mind.

Nothing that we are perceiving, remembering, or creating in brain is 'raw data'. Everything is colored (and sometimes manufactured) by our inner and outer state.

The question, then, bears repeating. Are your thoughts generally positive or negative? How do you 'take' the world around you?

Do you perceive predominantly:
- judgement?
- kindness?
- success?
- failure?
- challenge?
- opportunity?

Where do your thoughts lie when you truly pay attention? Sometimes the underlying mental pattern is camouflaged by learned behaviors.

What is really there? Why? Are your thoughts how you'd like them to be? And could they be stunting relationships, career, confidence, health, more?

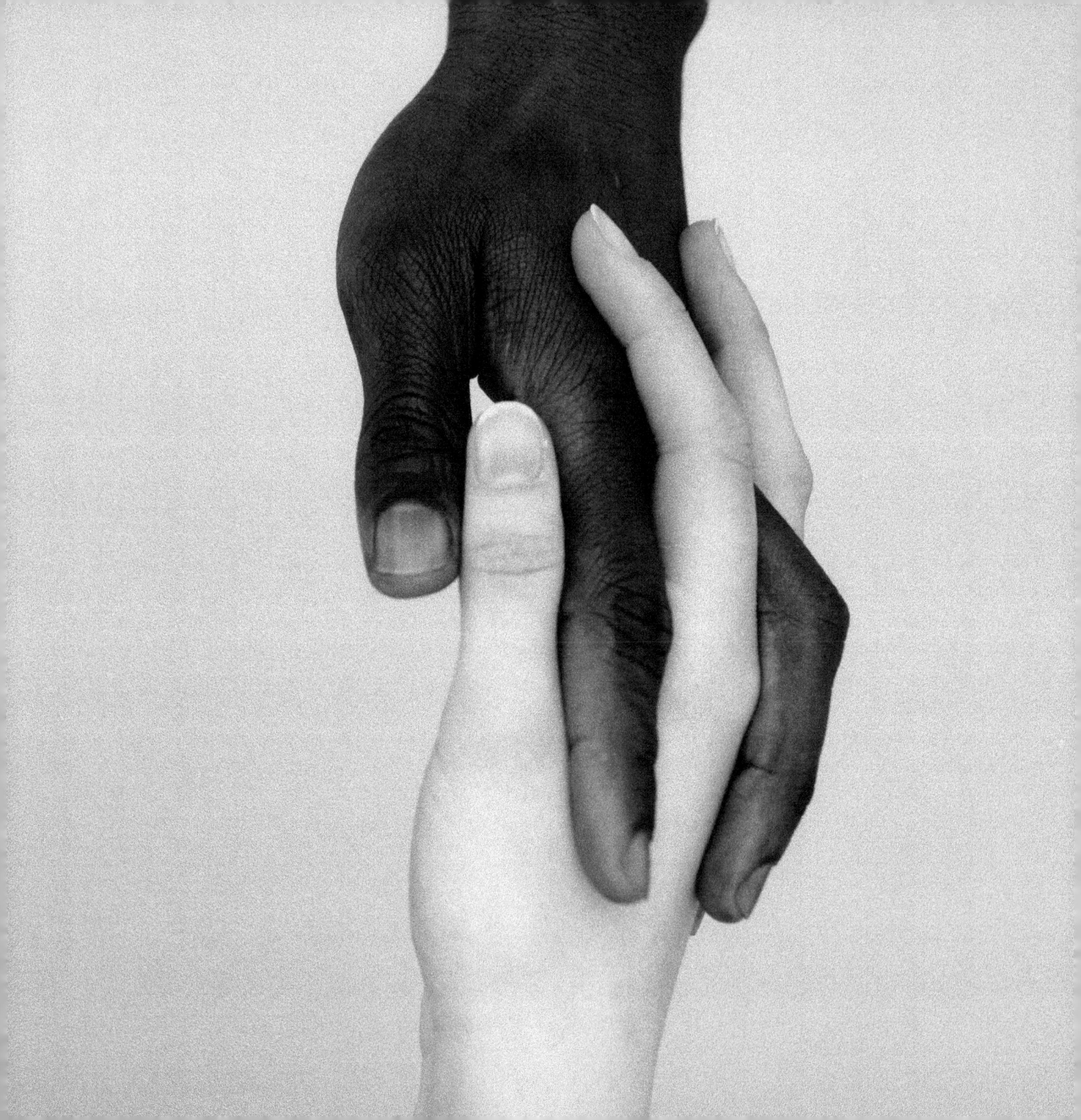

PREJUDICE

Wake up to your own, conscious or unconscious, prejudice(s).

You may be thinking to yourself:
- I've told the odd joke, but I don't really believe those generalizations.
- I only base my opinions on what I've seen or experienced—that's not prejudice.
- I have many BIPOC friends.
- I don't see color/I'm post-race.

Prejudice, according to Cambridge dictionary, is "an unfair and unreasonable opinion or feeling, especially when formed without enough thought or knowledge". All of the above statements may well apply to you. But search back in the annals of your memory.

It's time to be real with ourselves.

Imagine you happened to be born—that same spirit that is you—in another body, in a different country, with different genetics? With different customs and norms, different organizational structures and systems, different laws, freedoms, and barriers to access? Would you hold the same false notions about a particular group, race, age, or gender? Would others, born privileged, be right to judge you, your mother, your child?

It is not enough to abhor racism, to hate hate. Not having prejudice is passive, comfortable, and, quite frankly, nowhere near enough.

We need to be actively anti-racist. Actively anti-prejudice of any kind.

When will we wake up enough to see what we might unwittingly be perpetuating, via silence, ignorance, or both?

When will we awake to see that the only way to work toward true peace, toward true compassion, is by exerting ourselves (with only love in our hearts and hands) towards those ends?

Talk about getting mindful.

Let us all wake up.

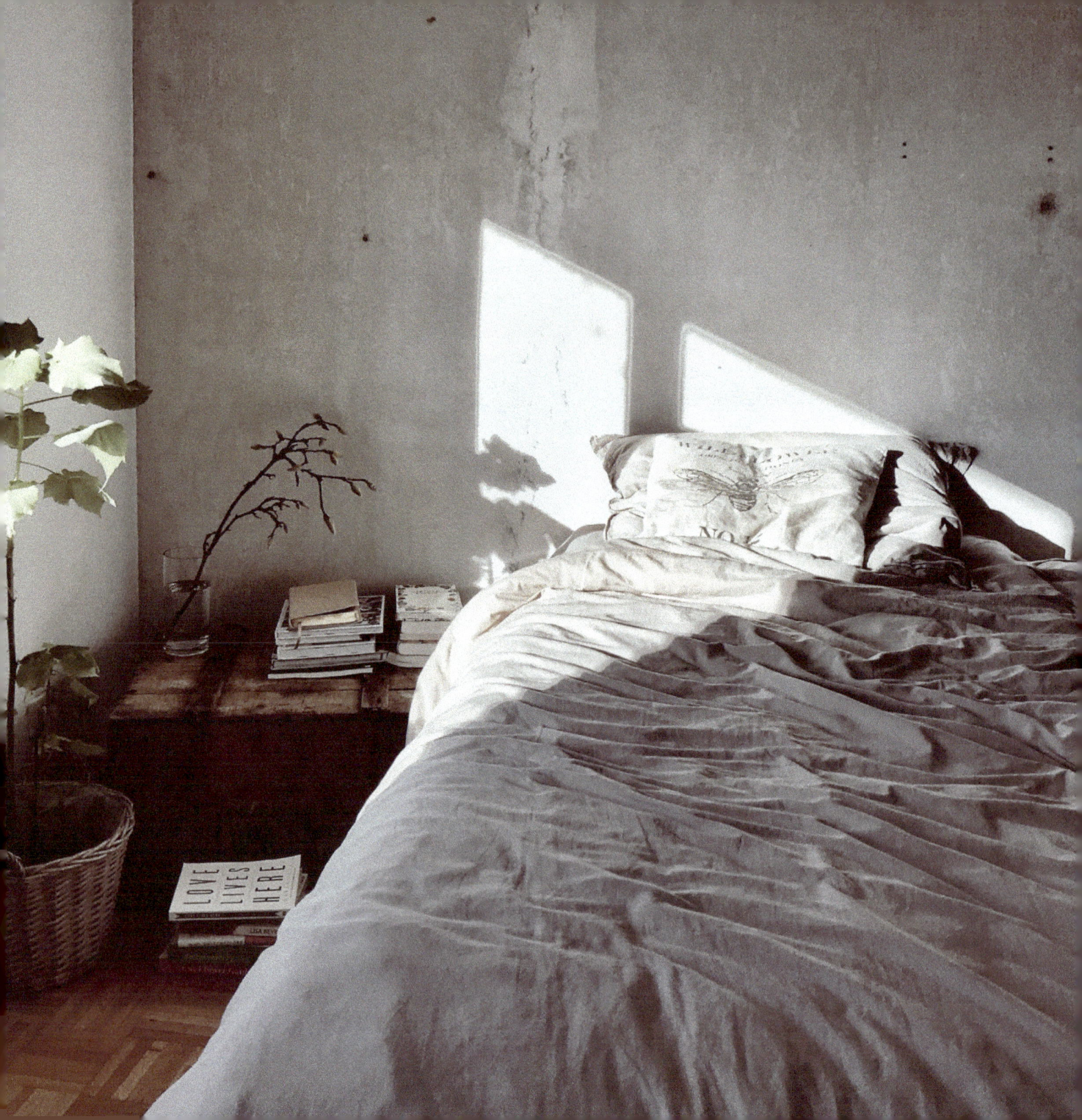

LOVE LIVES HERE

SLEEP

Wake up to your sleep.

Most of us are aware of the quality and quantity of our slumber. It's hard not to be, especially when it's in a state of lack.

Not to pour salt in the wound, but really everyone should know that poor sleep doesn't only affect your mood, energy levels, and patience (though these are undeniably crucial to our wellbeing). There are other, rather key, reasons to pay attention and start working towards optimizing your sleep. Over and above improving communication, emotional regulation, and mood, good sleep also:
- balances your immune system
- aids in weight loss (via leptin and insulin regulation)
- blunts sugar and carbohydrate cravings
- allows for tissue repair and recovery
- boosts muscle building and athletic performance
- increases productivity, focus, and memory
- detoxes chemicals in brain and body that build up throughout the day
- reinforces better sleep the next night and the ones thereafter (in a glorious positive loop)

How does the quantity and quality of your own sleep affect you? On nights where you've slept terribly, what happens to you the next day? Who do you lose it on? Is your self-talk louder, more judgmental?

Are you less productive at work or less attentive to your kids, or...?

Get to know precisely what disrupted or truncated sleep does to you specifically. By that same token, get to know you at your best—those times when you've slept like a baby—and see if you can pinpoint what you did differently to achieve this. Was it caffeine intake or timing? Food amounts, food types? No / less alcohol? Abstaining from media before bed? Morning exercise? Some form of decompression?

Whatever contributed, could it be reproduced?

This exercise in self-awareness is the most individualized health advice you could ever ask for. It's available, accessible, and free. Find resources on getting better sleep online, or go visit a naturopathic doctor who can tailor a plan for you. And then, friend, go and do something about that slumber.

Here's to soul-restoring sleep.

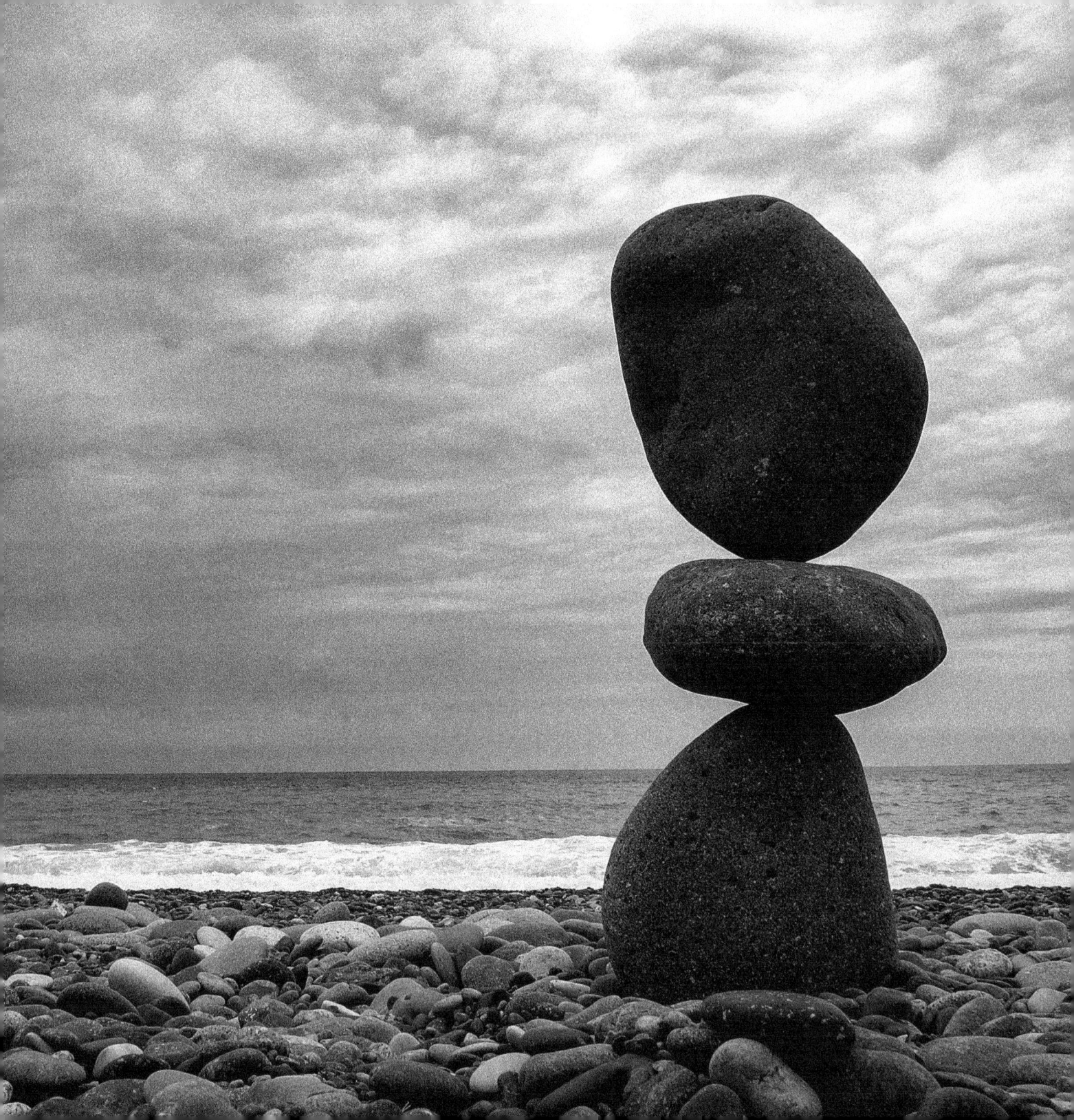

BALANCE

Wake up to Balance.

How can one word have become so incredibly cliché? In an age of self-help everything, we'd be hard pressed to find one article, book or podcast that hasn't mentioned it.

Of course, it is a concept that applies to so many aspects of our lives, there is not a singular definition. We are being told to "find balance" by our counsellors, our doctors, our partners, our best friends. And most of us are continually attempting some semblance of this in every aspect of our lives, however imperfectly. For the sake of building self-awareness, we need not actually achieve this balance, nor to even attempt to. Instead, it is to become acquainted with all the aspects of your life that may need a check-in.

Let go of any notion of balance as being an equal amount of dollar coins on either side of a scale. Instead, close your eyes and picture this:

A giant, old-school type scale the size of your backyard. Add anything you'd like to on either side (beach balls, pebbles, pool noodles, kitchen appliances, jewelry, books—anything). Take a few things off, add a few more on, until it levels out and settles. Ah, now here's a picture of true balance. We'll never be able to devote time or energies equally to all things and all people: this is simply an impossibility. Accepting this truth will largely prevent our own judgement and false feelings of failure.

You have not failed. For everything there is a season. If you're a new parent, your spirit will be rightly zeroed in and overtaken by all things baby and you. So, you take a bunch of items off the scale to counter-weigh the new responsibilities. A new love, a new job, learning a new skill, healing from an illness, or from grief? Apply this to every situation and adjust as necessary.

Now, become aware of what your scale looks like for the following situations:
- professional vs. personal time
- yourself vs. your family
- seriousness vs. play
- more nourishing foods vs. less nourishing foods
- waking vs. sleeping
- movement vs. stillness
- things you fight for vs. things you let go

Is there anything you'd like to add or take away to balance the scales? These efforts are continually in flux. If you're doing it imperfectly, you're doing it right.

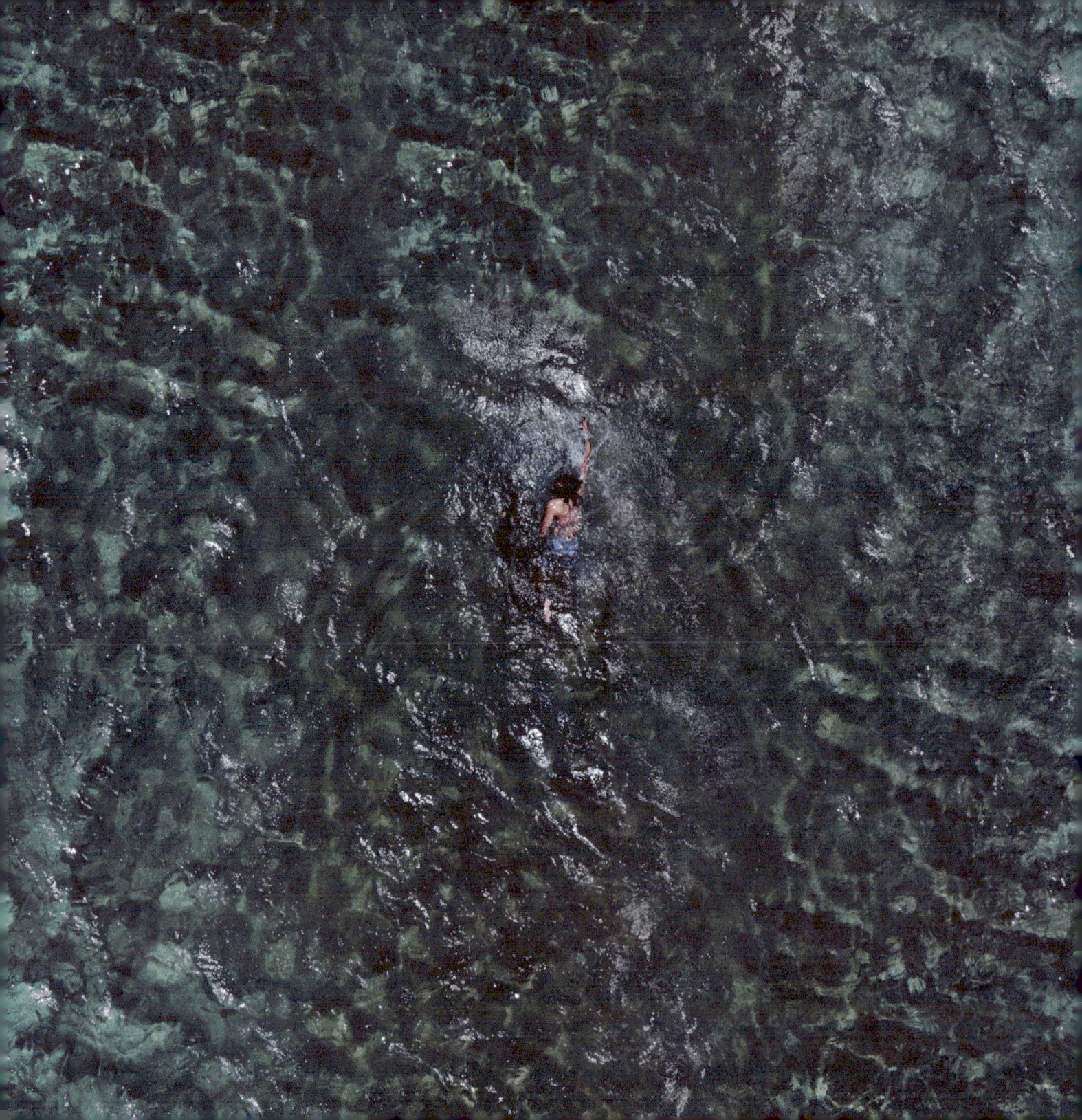

PACE

Wake up to your pace. Your daily pace, your life pace, that with which you normally engage in tasks—whether mundane or meaningful.

Are you:

1. Always on overdrive?
2. Performing some tasks as though an animal with its head cut off and others with great planning, attention, and care?
3. Always mega-mindful, having embraced the ethos of slow?

Chances are that most of us fall into one of the first two categories. Here's the truth: no matter how long or how deeply you've studied mindfulness or how many vipassana retreats you've attended, Western society dictates that we must *produce* and productivity and efficiency are golden skills in the workforce. When we use these traits to select for promotions and various enticing opportunities, the near reverence granted to them begins to spill over into our personal lives.

If we can just fit in that phone call while on our commute. If we can manage to squeeze that appointment in between clients. If we can cook dinner while scrolling social while writing out our grocery list. Well now *that* was a moment to feel proud of.

Check in. Where's your overall pace at? Does it match the ease/dis-ease, the rate/rhythm/character of your breath and pulse?

This is by no means a demonization of the appropriate and judicious use of efficiency and productivity. Instead, like the rest of the prompts in this section, it's a reminder to (at the very least) become aware of the ways in which they show up in your life, to what benefit, and what potential detriment.

Ironically, the simple act of bringing awareness to anything really does slow us down. It's no secret, I am consciously pushing us in that direction in this section of the book. And I'm doing so because I know we are so far off the rails in the other direction that we're in danger of missing out on so very much.

As we cross off to-do list tasks and realize we have barely spoken with our children, what feelings accompany? When we have sufficiently 'accomplished' the doing state at the expense of the being state, what kind of human_____ does that leave us?

What if we slowed down, just the tiniest bit, to see what we could see?

In all our rushing, what have we been missing?

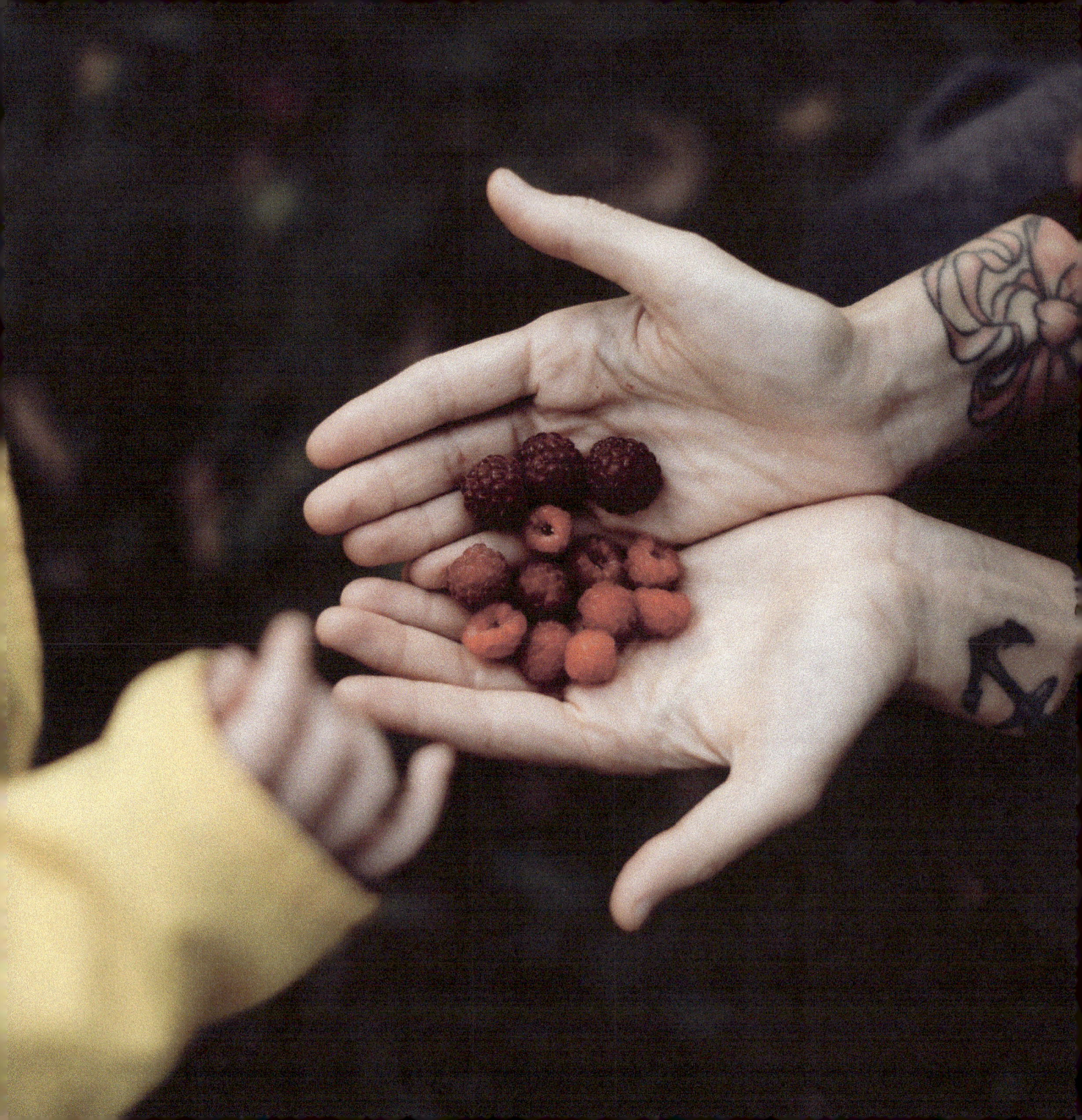

GRATITUDE

Wake up to gratitude.

Oh, rich, bountiful life. Which people, which moments, which elements do I take for granted? Take as given?

When we're asked to bring attention to what we're grateful for, often our brains go to one of two (positive) places:
- autopilot mentions like aspects of my
  health, my family, my work, the food on my table
- smaller moment-type responses like: "I'm grateful for the smooth ride into work this morning" or
"I'm grateful for that sweet exchange with my partner over breakfast"

Yes, these are things we must keep on our hearts and minds. But even when faced with significant difficulty, can we appreciate that hardship is also an appropriate, expected, vital aspect of life that is, in fact, responsible for new learnings, creation, and motivating positive changes? When we think that our struggles are not the way it's supposed to be, this thought creates a greater level of upset. We become increasingly focused on how hard everything seems to be for us; we become indignant, forgetting both that pain can serve us well and that there are likely oceans of treasure that we've forgotten the sight of. Oceans we're likely wading in at all times. Can we find gratitude for what has kept us alive, developing, falling and getting back up again? Can we do this without having to classify each experience with either a positive or negative valuation?

Close your eyes. Look at a typical day. Peek back to see what has led you to where you are, personally, professionally, spiritually. Can you place what elements had to be at play for that great thing to happen to you? Or for that crappy thing to happen so you could become better at something, more resilient? What was fundamental for you to develop the sheer skill, bandwidth, raw materials to enjoy any of the following?
- Getting a great job
  (or one that was a stepping stone to the great job)
- Having a family (starting one, keeping one, making one happy)
- Overcoming adversity
- Meeting a personal goal

What or who played a crucial role in the above? What was (amidst stress, being busy, being self-absorbed) never properly appreciated? We begin by envisioning the past as it's often easiest to see what came before, facilitated by time, distance, and perspective. We, of course, wouldn't be employing mindfulness if we didn't also look at our present day. Take stock of where and how you are today. Now ask: Why? Why, what things, which people, which aspects of life continue to allow this or that thing to run smoothly for me? Take stock of each wave, of each ripple, as you practice. Have gratitude for the pleasant and unpleasant things that have been overlooked.

Go deep. And go daily.

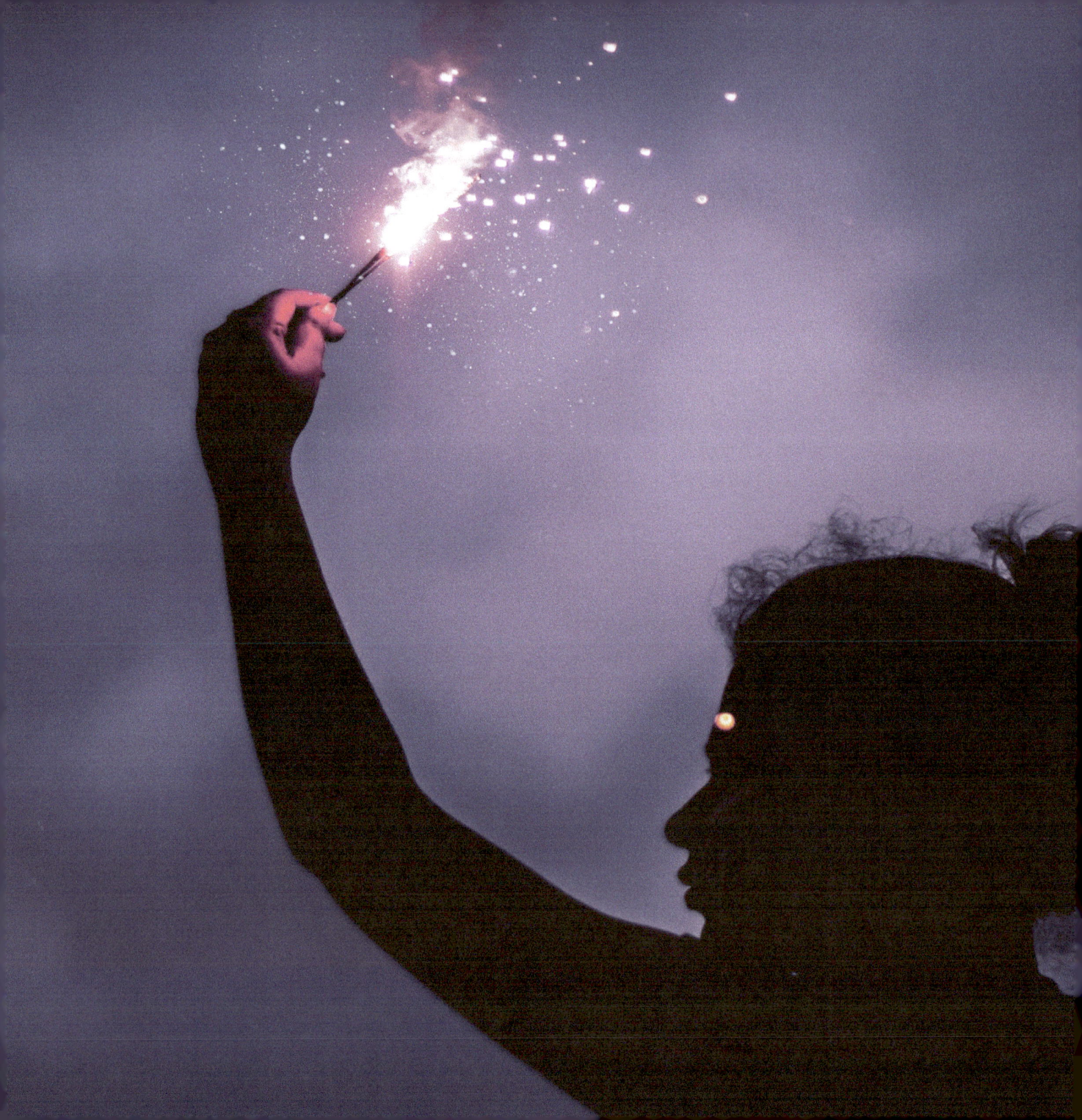

TRIGGERS

Wake up to what aggravates you.

We usually think of aggravating factors in the form of people: our boss, coworker, in laws, etc.

In naturopathic medicine, when we talk about aggravation and alleviation, we're referring to those elements that make our condition worse or better, respectively. In short, triggers are those factors that (reliably) make us feel worse. Symptom x flares when we eat this food or this category of food. Symptom y goes off the charts when we repress emotion/consume caffeine/have fitful sleep, etc. You get the picture.

When I see patients for the first time, a big part of our discussion is regarding "obstacles to cure". What proverbial ragweed are you walking through daily that is preventing you from proper healing, no matter what other healthful changes you are making? And though some triggers may be obvious to us, others are elusive.

Awareness, as we've been attempting to hone through the prompts in this section (and which meditation and mindfulness practices do such powerful work to support) is not always immediately or easily accessible. It takes actual noticing *work,* however simple. Over time, we build a picture. We begin to see patterns. When nine times out of ten eating or drinking whatever-it-is precipitates an aggravation, the trigger (and your agency in the matter) is revealed.

Are you in touch with all that ails you? If so, are you following that up with actions that align?

Or could you be paying more attention to the things you do, the foods you consume, the rest you get, the interactions you engage in…?

Becoming aware gifts us the absolute clearest and most compelling evidence with which to guide how we are to heal ourselves.

Know the offending allergen, cure the allergy.

We can only successfully use an arrow if we can have its target in view.

IMPATIENCE

Patience/impatience is a spectrum. On the line joining both ends, there is a slider that moves along it in either direction and is always moving, back and forth—faster or slower—depending on our underlying mood, our sleep, our nutrition, and how many times we've been faced with that particular hurdle.

It's empowering to realize that patience, too, can be strengthened via a dedicated mindfulness practice. So strengthened, in fact, that instead of being wholly subject to the whims of our sleep, our children's tantrums, or the stressors at work, it becomes resistant to those things. They become extraneous.

Think of the various ways your inner or outer state are currently affected by external factors. Wouldn't it be a significant strength to have more control over that slider? To feel certain that a difficult interaction with someone would see a calm, consistently patient you showing up to greet it, regardless of the climate of your life that day?

Being affected by impatience is not all bad. Growing impatient with a job or goal can help us look for alternatives that might be more worthwhile.

At times, it can help get us out of a rut of singular thinking that has caused us to be blind to more favorable options. Like most stress, it's not so much its presence in our lives, but how we react to it that makes all the difference.

Still, when we are full to the brim with decision fatigue, with an unending rolodex of options, with a waning work ethic, that old virtue—patience—would sure be useful. Strengthening it would help us work harder to reach our goals, push us to see them to their ends and to truly appreciate the results of our efforts and our time. This is essentially why the acquisition of trainers, coaches and accountability buddies has become quite so ubiquitous.

We need a sensei of sorts to watch over and force us to kick another one hundred times. Or to stop yelling… until we get it.

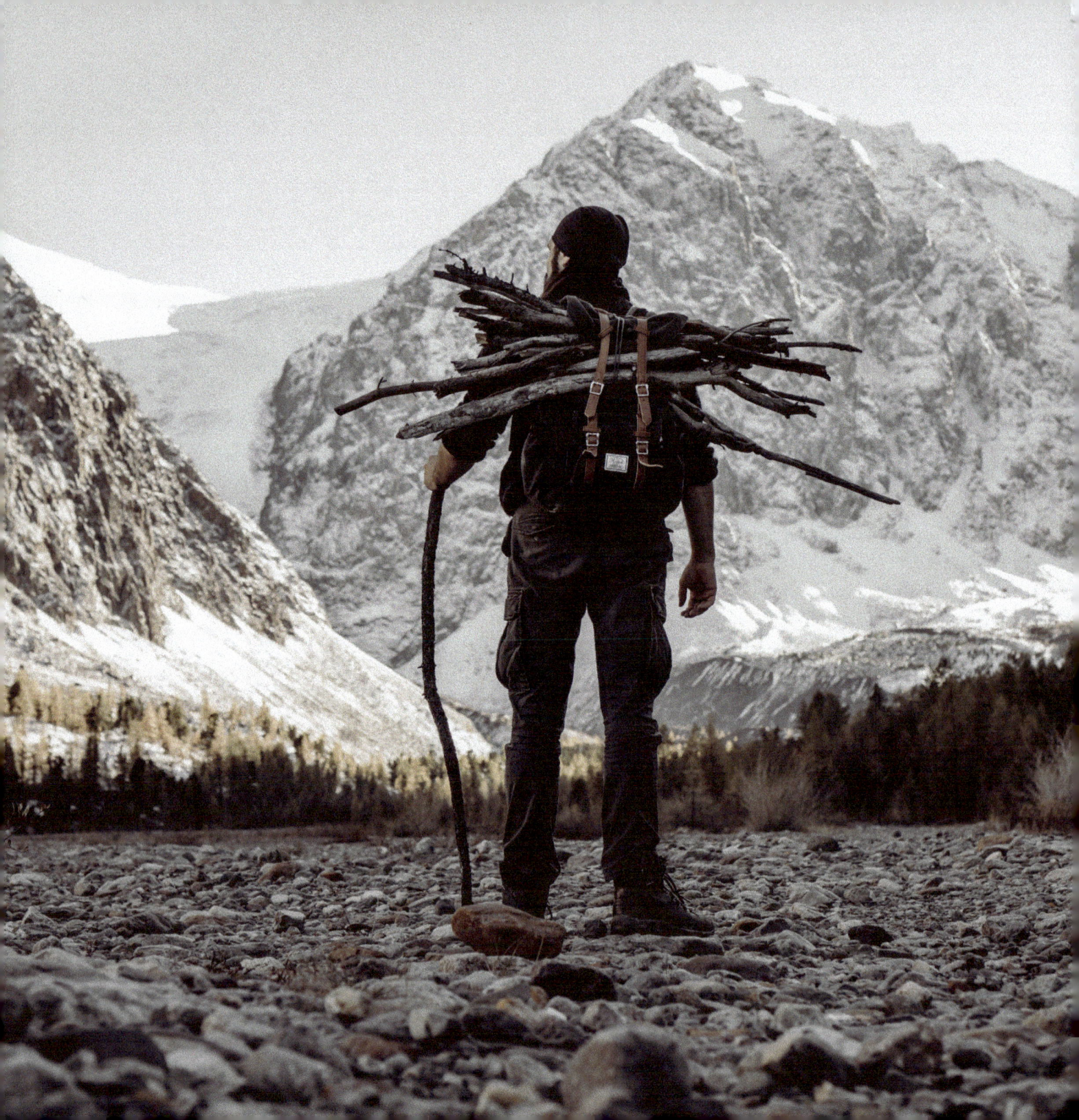

STRENGTHS

Wake up to your strengths.

In the world of self-development, we love placing emphasis on breaking ego like a shattered window and fessing up, to ourselves if not to others, in all the ways we're lacking. Have you, along your betterment journey, become aware of the fact that you are a workaholic? Or less than mindful with your spouse or kids? Or do you eat too much junk or exercise too much? Do you gossip or lie? Are you a people pleaser or super selfish?

While it's undoubtedly useful and necessary to be able to fully see how we are and what we present to those around us, it's also true that, like all things, this lacks moderation and balance. Have you been beating yourself up far too much?

Depression is a serious, widespread, and largely underdiagnosed problem. Often the notion that we are not enough or that we have no good to share is at its root.

Just for a moment, try to answer this: What are your superpowers? Yes, plural. Is one making restaurant-quality food for you and your family? Is it being world class at remembering birthdays or other days of significance? Maybe it's your sense of humor or a physical skill? Did you co-create and/or birth a human? Do you make beautiful art? Are you the best listener?

Whatever it is that's uniquely you and great about you, become aware of all of it. What qualities would your best friend list about you if asked what makes you amazing? If you really have no idea, then, please, outright ask them. You deserve to know what makes you special to them.

It's also a great idea to journal out the ways in which you see yourself as remarkable. Some of us will find this easy, others will be hard pressed to utter or write a word in this vein. Truly, beyond how society has labeled you or how you've labeled yourself, what strengths lie within?

Once you've got a few nuggets of gold, allow yourself one sweet moment of relish. Swim in that pool like Uncle Scrooge McDuck, wading through his dollar bills.

Allow yourself to remember the ways in which you are strong and wonderful.

Exceptionally you.

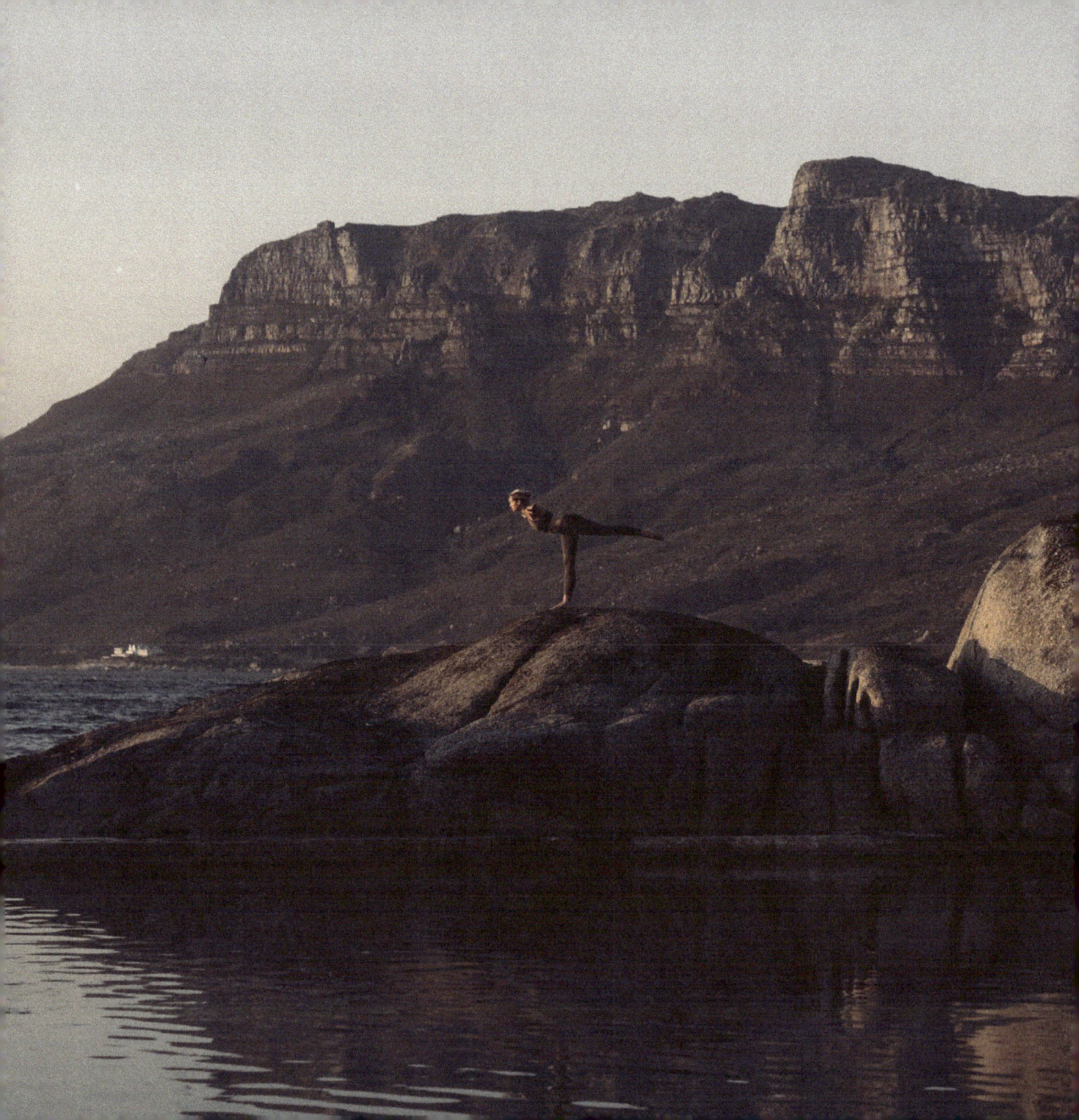

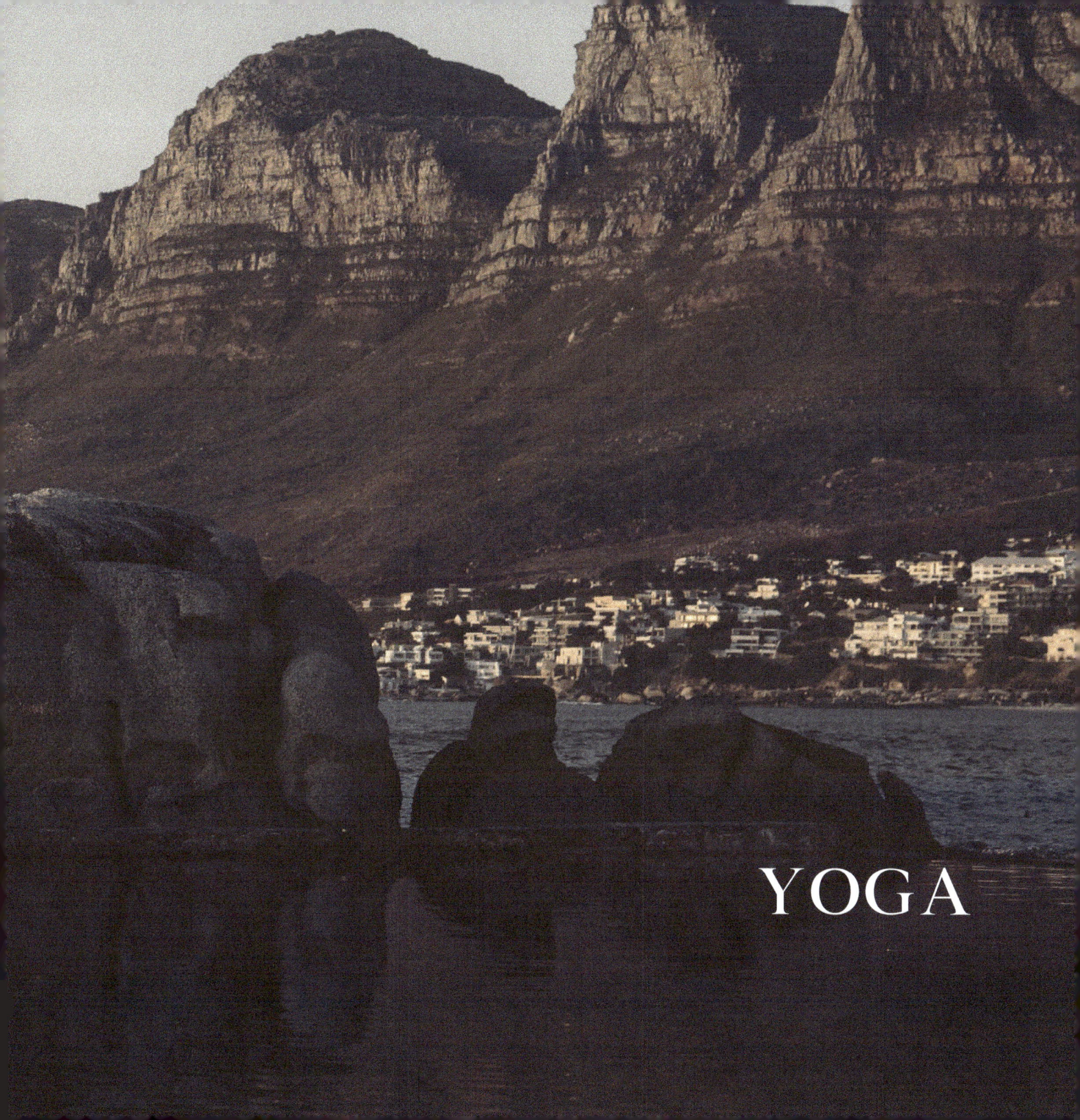

YOGA

WHAT YOGA ISN'T

If you've practiced yoga outside of its regions of origin, chances are you entered a class in a studio, and there, an instructor guided you through a series of poses. This likely included some emphasis on the breath. It may or may not have included a very short meditation, depending on the teacher's training, lineage, or leaning.

The postures are called asana. Asana can change our bodies and our minds. They can increase flexibility, strength, stamina, balance, self-awareness. They can ease pain. They can open us, physically and emotionally.

Their primary purpose, however, is to prepare us for sitting—sitting with a strong back, relaxed shoulders, flexible, open hips and knees, a mind that is not racing. We can, rather acutely, appreciate this preparation when shifting our bodies from standing or chair-sitting, to sitting cross-legged on a flat surface for long periods of time.

The practice of asana, however, is not the whole of yoga. There are many texts already written describing the various components of this multifaceted practice (which only partially include controlled breathwork and meditation) and I'll refer you, dear reader, to any number of those books and articles to learn more about yoga's other "limbs."

It's important to understand that when most of us in the West discuss yoga, we are generally referring to only that which goes on within the walls of the studio, primarily, the practice of the physical postures. For the purposes of this book (and for sake of clarity), I will be using the term yoga to reference this aspect of the practice. Know that it is a partial definition only.

Though there is far more, the postural elements are so very worthy of study and, in and of themselves, have the power to change our lives.
Let's start here.

One library at a time.

[While I consider all of the postures that follow to carry a definite "magic," there is nothing exceptional about these as compared to other postures that were not included in this book. The following is a random sampling of poses—some seated, some standing—each requiring more or less flexibility, balance, strength, etc. than another, but all requiring equal amounts of practice, attention and breath. I've begun the section with Mountain and ended it with Corpse, as many structured classes tend to do. Other than this, the asana included are special for their unique challenges and benefits, though not more or less so than the many, many beautiful poses not highlighted here.]

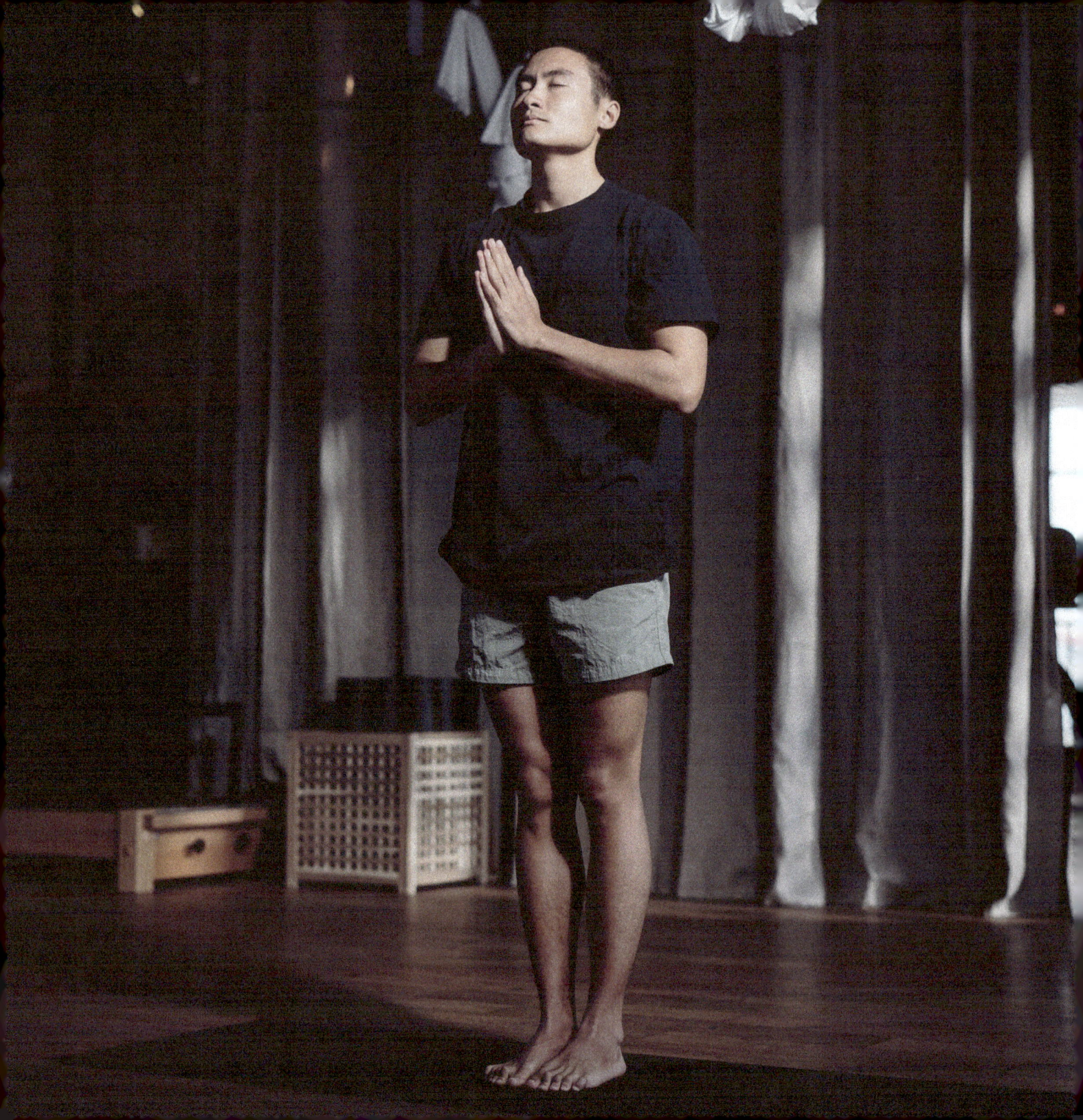

TADASANA - MOUNTAIN POSE

OFF the Mat:

Standing. We tend to see this as an easy, nothing-much-to-do pose. We want to get on with it and arrive at harder challenges. If you are truly in Tadasana, after following all the tips below (and I could have gone on forever), are you doing nothing? Is it easy to keep track of all of it, in a relaxed but strong way, alongside natural, flowing breath?

What other aspects or moments of your life are like the Mountain? There is no easy pose. All is effort. And all effort yields reward.

Tadasana:
- helps the body/spine to regain proper posture
- stands us upward to counter the ever-downward process of age and time
- works the mind to seek physical balance in a way that we rarely give attention to when out-of-pose standing. (Are we ever truly centered, not leaning too far forward or too far back? Have you ever noticed?)

ON The Mat:

- Knees face forward, energetically pull knees and quads upward
- Weight is resting on the center (arches) of your feet with even pressure on balls of feet and heels; teeter back and forth between those until you find a happy medium
- Eyes look softly forward

- Think of pulling the back of the head slightly up in space so your chin tucks in a bit, lengthening the back of your neck
- Have all the natural curvatures of the spine intact, spinal column aligned (avoid hyperextending or flexing)
- Shoulders down, relaxed and aligned over hips
- Lower abdominals pull in and upward, sternum raised
- Visualize standing tall, powerful, strong—resistant to whatever environment surrounds you (you know, like a mountain)

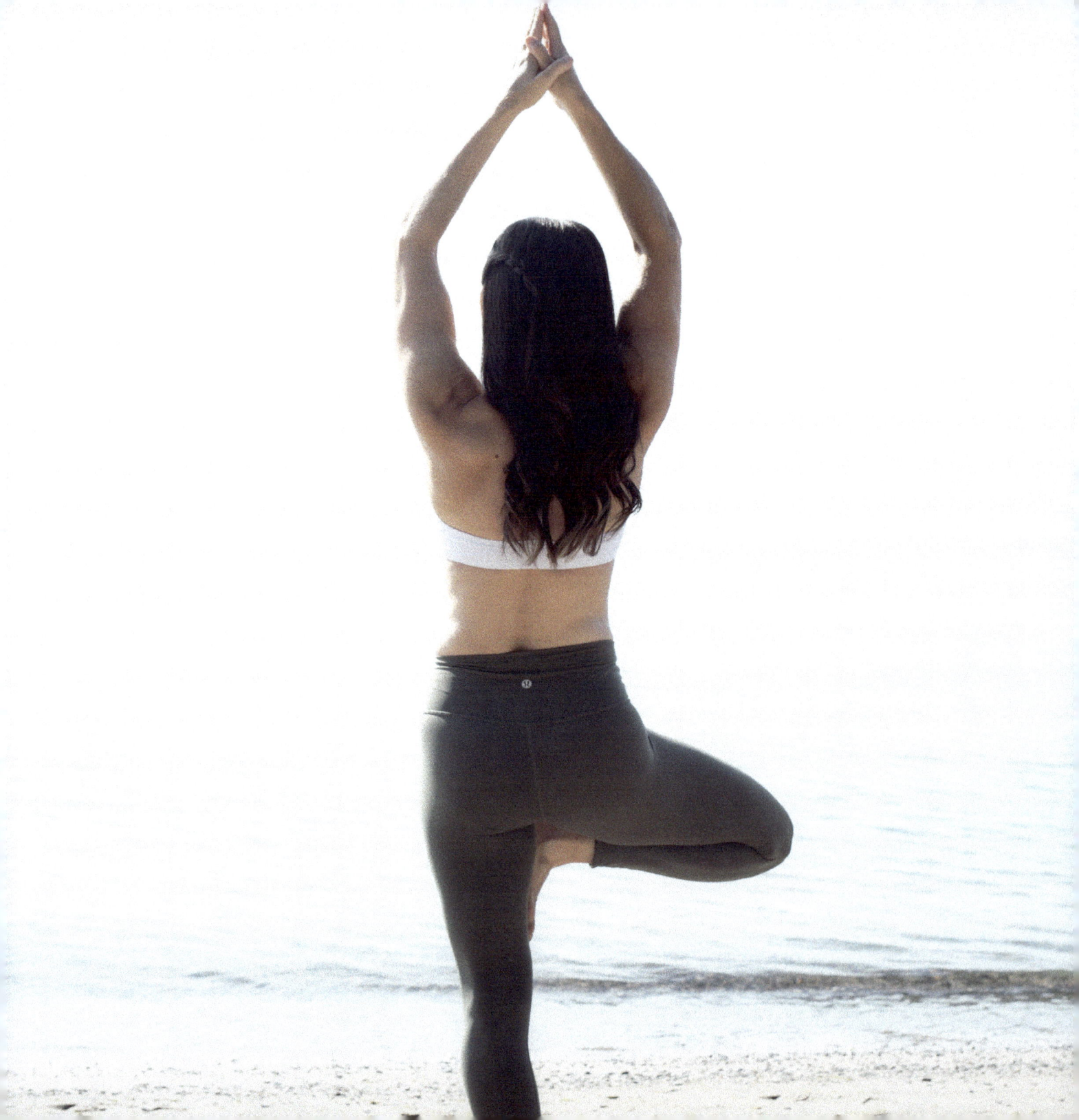

VRKSASANA - TREE POSE

OFF the Mat:

- Improves focus/concentration, proprioception
- Cultivates equanimity (mental calm, composure, even temper throughout difficulty)
- Grounds us when life feels turbulent—brings us in touch with the understanding that the tree's strength in staying upright and intact through gales lies in its *give*, in its flexibility, in its ability to sway in the wind without losing rootedness

* With a strong and steady mind, there is no wind nor storm you cannot weather gracefully

ON the Mat:

- Find a gentle point of focus (called a drishti, or "yogic gaze") across from you
- Use your standing leg to push down strongly into the earth and feel the equal and opposite force from the earth back into your standing leg (we get back what we put in)
- Lifted foot is to be actively pressing into the inner calf or thigh of the standing leg, avoid pushing into the knee joint
- The bent knee moves as outwardly (laterally) as your physical structure allows. We have different bodies; not only flexibility, but skeletal/muscular structure as well. Though, with practice, you will always evolve in a posture (the more your body will open), we have to also get to know our bodies and accept their structural limitations.

KEY: Both hip bones face straight forward, pelvis is even. Hips should be just as square and balanced as though in standing/Mountain pose.

- Belly draws in toward the spine, core engaged
- Hands can be in prayer in front of you, lifted in prayer above you, opened to shoulder distance above you and swaying, behind you in reverse prayer (anything so long as shoulders are relaxed, down and away from the ears)
- You may develop such strong stability that you can start lifting your gaze to the sky
- Tuck your chin in slightly to lengthen the back of the neck

Wobbling, leaning, falling out of the pose—these are all welcomed. All of them will happen and will change every time you step onto the mat (use this pose to get a feel for where you are today).

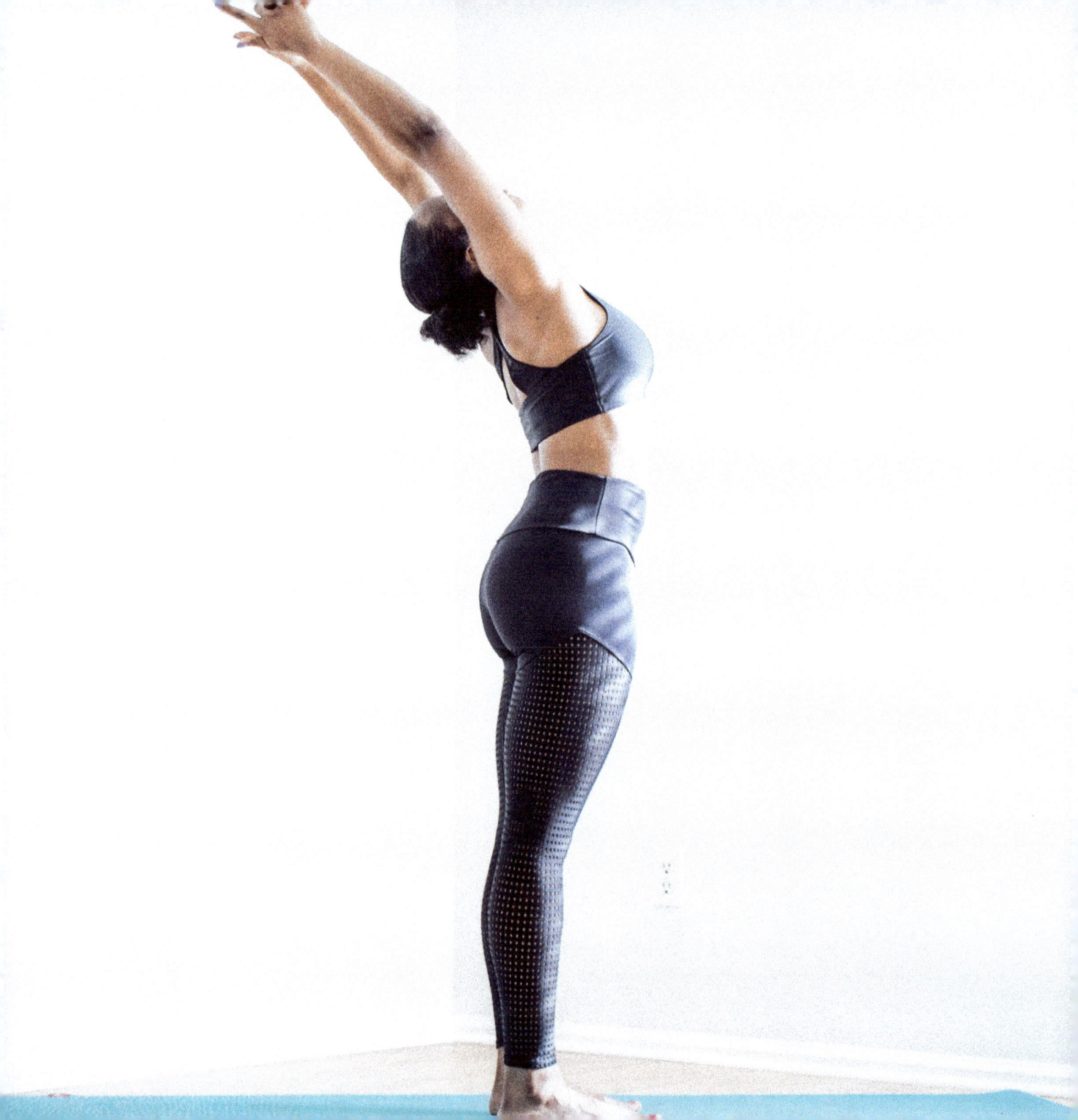

ANUVITTASANA - STANDING BACKBEND POSE

OFF the Mat:

Like any pose that involves back bending / bringing your chest up and forward...this is a heart opener. This allows us to:

- introspect, check in: can you let go of any resistance toward someone hard to love, hard to accept? Can you open your heart to you?
- experience and strengthen empathy and compassion

In time, holding this pose for many breaths at a time will open the muscles that assist healthy respiration. It will also undo the front body guarding patterns created and nourished by frequent defensive ways of being (which, in turn, cause shallow, erratic breathing in a vicious cycle). When we backbend—when we heart-open—we break ourselves free and move purposefully into the world, with confidence and compassion. As we do, our breath (and thus our mind) becomes regular, rhythmic, deep...and calm.

ON the Mat:

- First, establish a strong Mountain pose and keep the engagement of the legs throughout, toes forward
- With shoulders rolled back, three options for arms: bring palms to back 'pockets' with fingers down, have them at heart center in prayer, or lift arms so biceps are beside ears (if you have shoulder concerns you may need to practice with arms lowered and hands behind)
- If arms are stretched above you, hands can remain shoulder width apart or fingers interlaced with index fingers released
- Keep the integrity of the hips and pelvis, framed forward, yet not jutting forward (you are still standing—hips should track mostly over the knees and knees over ankles in the same way)
- Tailbone is slightly tucked under
- Abdominals engaged
- Keeping the spine long, begin to lift up first and notice a slight arch backward when you do so—remember you are *opening the heart*: lift the sternum as though a string tied to it is pulling vertically toward the sky
- This requires engagement of the muscles of your neck. Look forward until the arch in your upper back has you looking upward, the back of neck should stay long and toned throughout.
- Shoulders stay down and away from the ears

As always, the right pose for you is the frame where you can breathe with ease. If you cannot do so, bring it back.

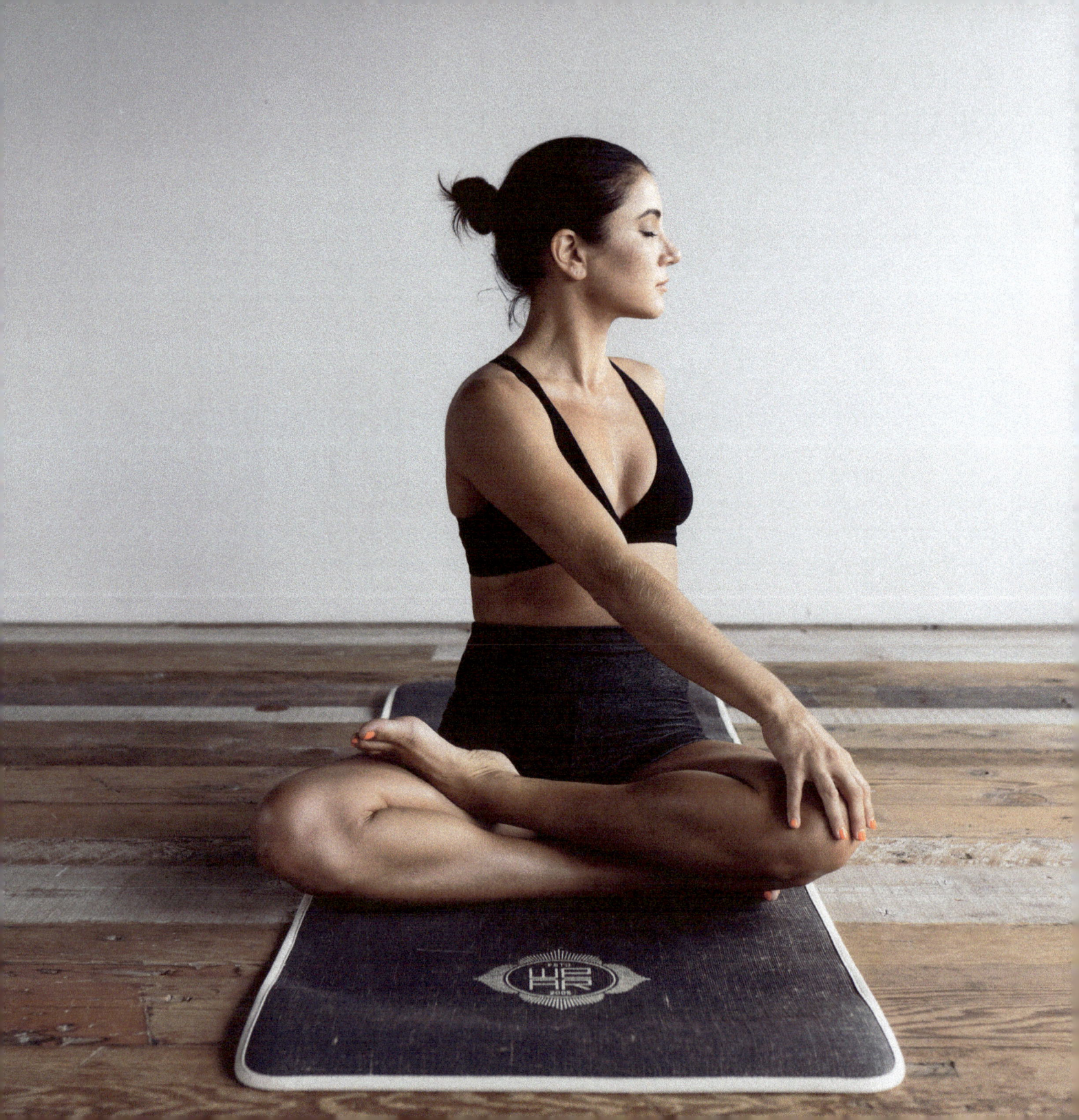

PARIVRTTA ARDHA PADMASANA - REVOLVED HALF LOTUS POSE

OFF the Mat:

Twists place pressure on the internal organs, often making a once easeful breath, a bit labored or constricted. A focused breath practice is helpful in achieving full inhales and exhales (which, when used in twists specifically, is a great way to exercise the respiratory muscles and increase lung capacity). What else in your life can you bring this full, easeful breath to, even when in distress? It's not ok to hold your breath until the pose or the tough time has passed. In fact, your wise body won't let you do that for long. In yoga, we know our proper place in the pose by using our breath as a gauge.

Notice the rate, rhythm, and depth of your breath as you walk through a stressful moment. Are there holding patterns? Is there shallowness or struggle? Practice this pose and note what it teaches.

- Brings fresh circulation to the entire spine, internal organs, and pelvis
- Opens the chest and ribs
- Re-aligns and strengthens the shoulder girdle
- Improves flexibility in the hips, knees, and ankles
- Aids digestion and healthy elimination

ON the Mat:

- Make sure your hips and knees are warmed up and open before beginning
- Sit with legs straight out in front of you
- Bend L knee, hug it into you and bring that ankle toward the R hip
- Sole faces up, top of foot nestled in the hip crease
- Sitting upright, lengthen the spine, making space between each vertebra. Think about grounding down equally with both sitting bones to reach upward through the spine.
- Place R hand over L knee, and gently press L hand into floor behind L hip (without sacrificing the integrity of your collarbones; keep these in one straight line)
- Begin to slowly twist your upper body to the L, keeping your neck in line with your spine. There is no use twisting your head to look way out over your shoulder if it brings it out of alignment. Ensure that everything above the hips moves together as if one unit, and that the hips and everything below remain facing forward. Engage the slightest rightward twist of the hips in order to keep them in place. It's a spinal twist, not solely a cervical one. Honesty in the pose.
- Take care not to lean forward nor press into your hands too hard
- Breathe
- Return to the center, and switch sides

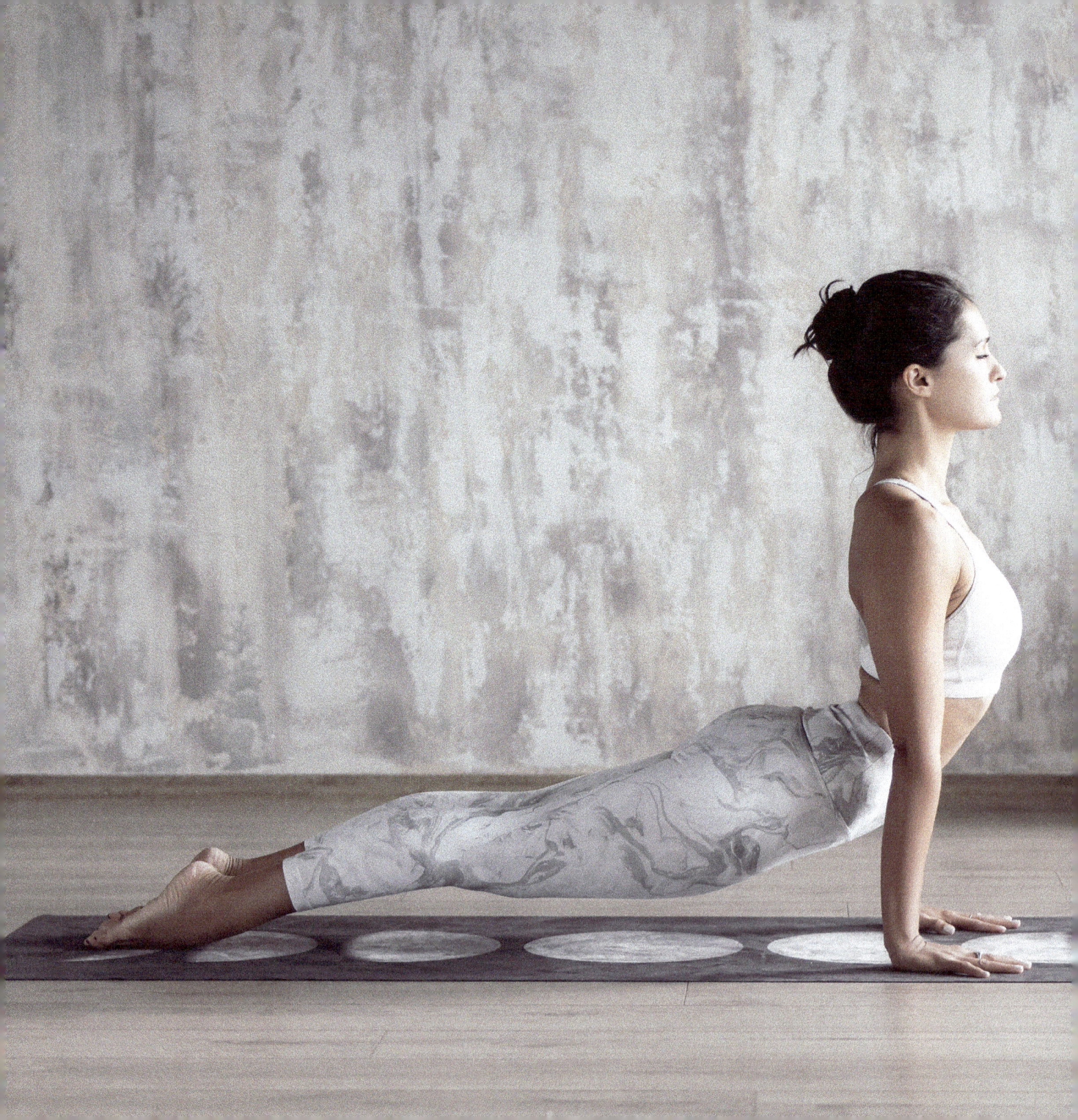

URDHVA MUKHA SVANASANA - UPWARD FACING DOG POSE

OFF the Mat:

In Traditional Chinese Medicine, the front body is considered yin (vulnerable, soft, feminine) and the back body is considered yang (energetic, masculine)

Sitting at a desk all day or using a phone or computer for hours is a common cause of slumping shoulders and poor posture. It follows that our moods are usually overwhelmed or depressed. Check your body: heart (and vulnerability) in and moving backward, protected.

Upward Facing Dog Pose is said to counter these states of depression and overwhelm by opening the front body and bringing the heart forward and confidently into the world.

[This pose is commonly used in the Surya Namaskar (sun salutation) sequence, and is the more yang, hips-lifted, option usually offered in place of Bhujangasana (Cobra pose)]

ON the Mat:

- Begin laying on the mat, belly and face down
- Hands flat under the shoulders
- Ground the tops of feet (so they are untucked) and bring the heels together
- As you lift your hips and knees off the floor, quadriceps and abdominals are fully engaged
- Pressure should be at the base of the fingers, shoulders aligning directly over wrists. Make sure palms are fully sealed to the floor.
- Tops of shoulders are way down and away from ears (the opposite of shrugging)
- Slight micro-bend in the elbows (eyes of the elbows forward, as though in plank)
- Though many yogis practice this pose with the neck extended backward and eyes facing the sky, proper alignment principles are what we're looking for: eyes forward, neck neutral, chin level with floor or slightest chin tuck as though pushing the back of your head into a wall behind you. Shoulder blades are to be kissing (picture the fronts of your shoulders rotating outward as though squeezing them together onto your back). Think: "heart softening forward" versus "throat forward".

* The hips-down version of this, called Bhujangasana (Cobra pose), can also be practiced without any arm strength or pressure in the hands at all. As a variation, prepare in the same way as above, hands under shoulders. Instead of initiating the movement with the press of hands, strongly engage the core, the muscles lining the spinal column as well as the legs and glutes to bring the torso up and forward. This will result in a much smaller movement of the upper body, but this pose is in no way smaller.

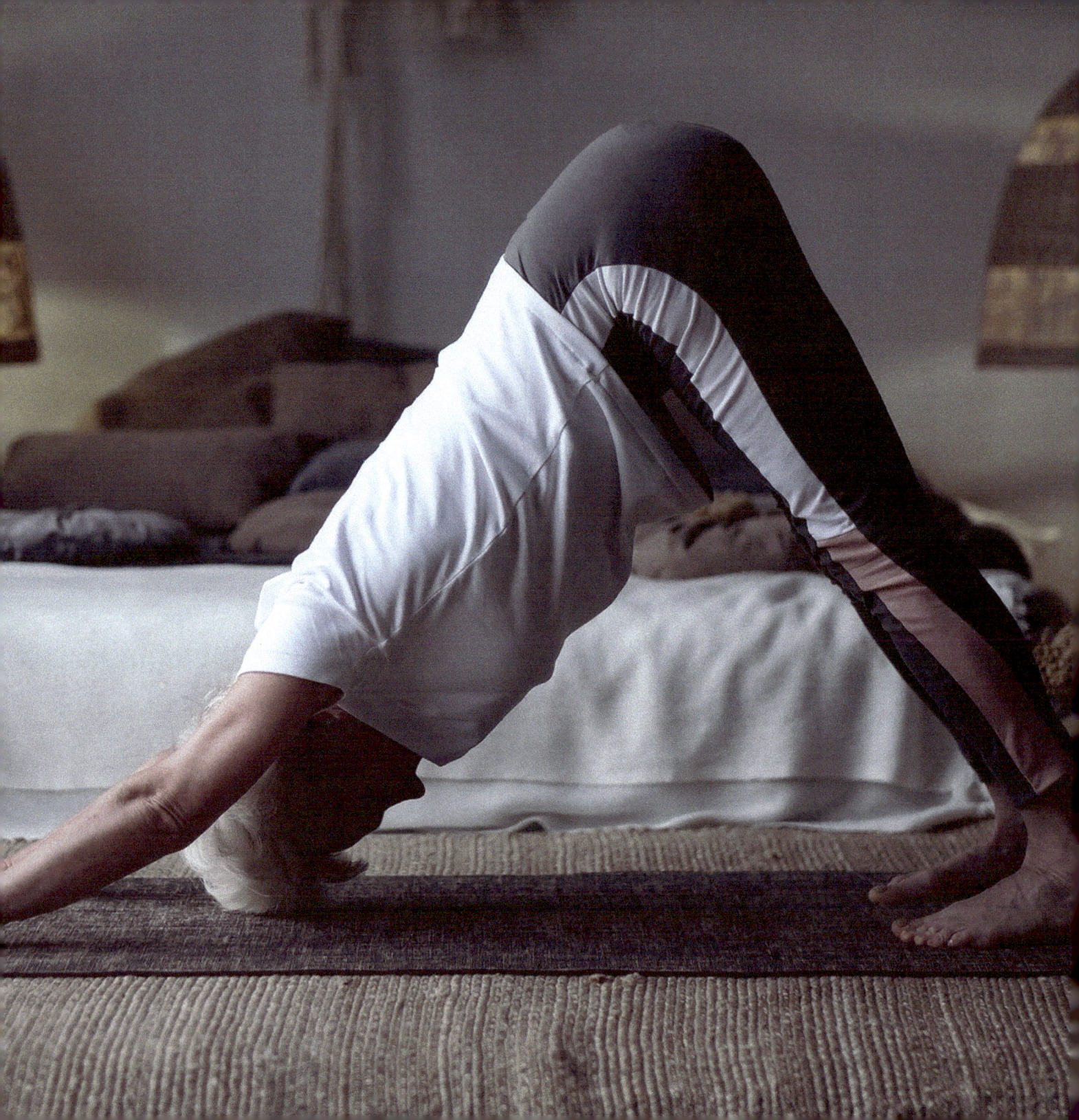

ADHO MUKHA SVANASANA - DOWNWARD FACING DOG POSE

OFF the Mat:

- Restores energy when fatigued
- Gently stimulates the nervous system
- Calms the brain as the head is lowered toward the Earth
- Brings the body and mind back to neutral, back to its home base (if you notice it sprinkled throughout most yoga classes, again and again, this is why)

Like many poses, on the surface this seems simple and easy. In fact, it's quite layered and complex when you break down everything that is going on. Try holding it (and all the alignment principles outlined below) for more than a minute and see how it calls us to stay present.

ON the Mat:

- Hands planted at the top of the mat, all four corners of the palms grounded, especially the pads at the base of the fingers (fingertips should be lightly on the mat, check they are not gripping)
- Let your hands push away from the Earth
- Feet begin parallel and remain so throughout the pose
- It's not important for your heels to be able to reach the ground (remember, different bodies, different flexibilities), but do let this be the intention of the heels—toward ground

KEY: The movement actually begins with the hips moving upward and backward in space. As though someone in front of you is gently pushing your sacrum toward the back of your mat while tilting your pelvis/sitz bones up and back

- Shoulder blades go down the back towards your hips: As you are inverted, this will look to an observer as your shoulder blades moving "up" towards the sky (this can be a tricky concept in practice...try to release the shrug, so the tops of the shoulders move away from the ears and bring your elbows slightly in so the head can relax somewhat. It's as though you are wrapping your shoulder blades around the back of your ribcage).
- Bring your heart up away from the ground and toward your legs
- Draw your belly in and up
- Your gaze is also back toward your legs, or to your belly button
- Breathe

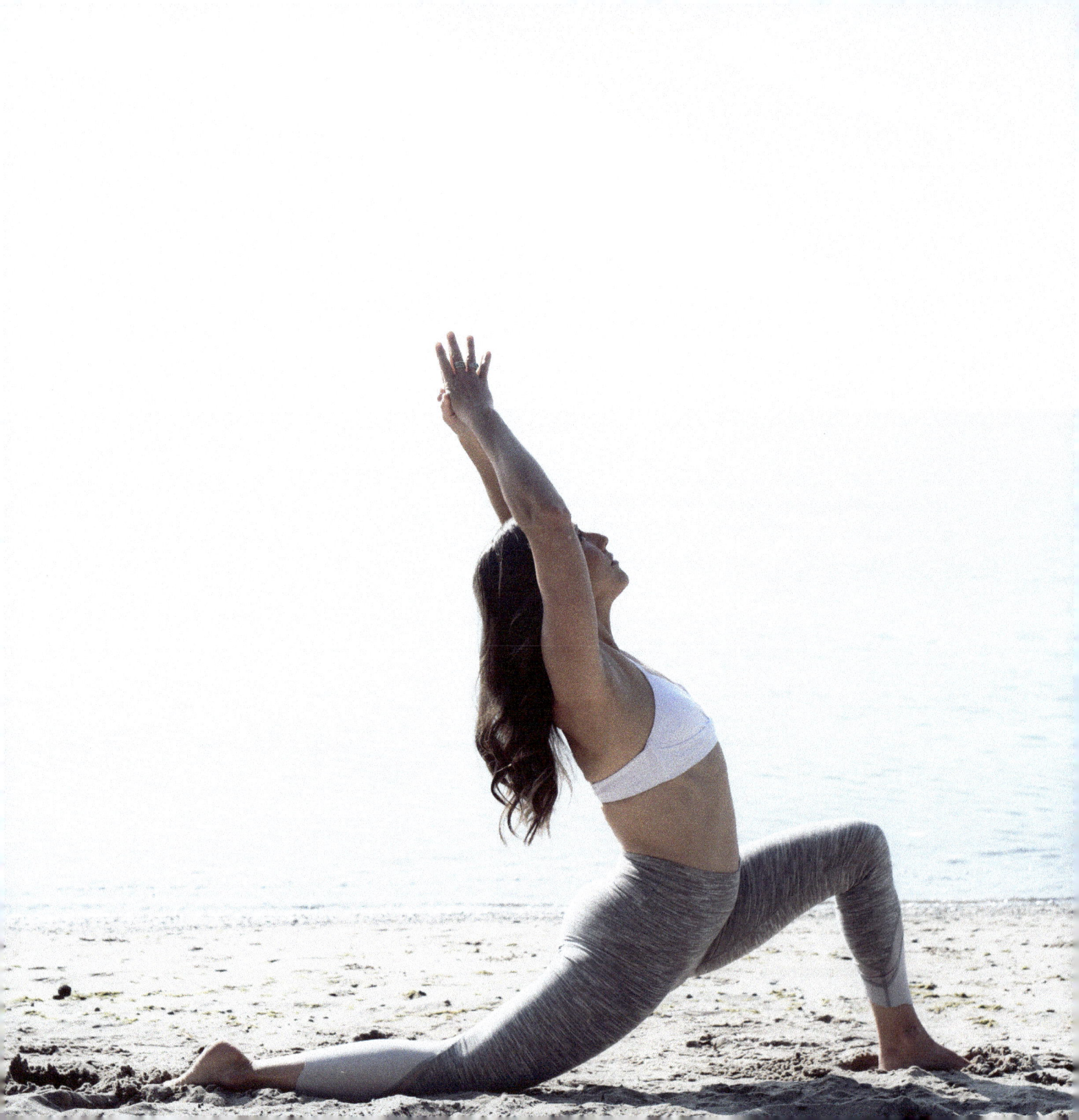

ANJANEYASANA -
LOW LUNGE / CRESCENT MOON POSE

OFF the Mat:

- Expands chest, lungs, and shoulders to help with breathing
- Builds coordination, concentration, and attention
- Strengthens balance: vertically, horizontally, in and out—where else might you apply this beautiful duality?

This pose allows us to ground deeply while at the same time rising up—so we root firmly with our bodies and minds, connecting with Earth strongly and, in so doing, uplift our spirit.

ON the Mat:

- The front foot is flat on the ground between your hands, hands can be flat on the ground (tent the fingertips if necessary) or arms raised in a slight backbend, as pictured here
- The front knee is directly over top the ankle
- Belly in, core engaged to protect the lower back
- As always, neck is in alignment with the spine (if in the slight backbend version, take care to not drop the head backward, always supporting the head with the muscles of the neck)
- The back knee stays planted on the mat behind you, far enough back that you feel an elongation in both the groin and hip flexors of the back leg as well as in the hamstrings and glutes of the front leg. The toes are untucked so that the top of the foot is resting on the ground.
- The idea is to scissor your legs energetically... You strengthen the muscles required to pull the front hip back in space and the back hip forward, without much visible movement at all
- Slightly tuck the pelvis under (if this concept is challenging, think of using the abdominal muscles to gently bring together the fronts of the hip bones towards the bottom ribs). Again, an observer would notice very little change here. With this fluid structure, gently glide your hips forward and down.
- Whether your hands are planted or raised to the sky in a crescent variation, shoulders are always down away from the ears
- Stay buoyant: The sensation is one of lengthening the lower body while holding a confident, upward energy.
- Once you've had many slow breaths here, repeat on the other side

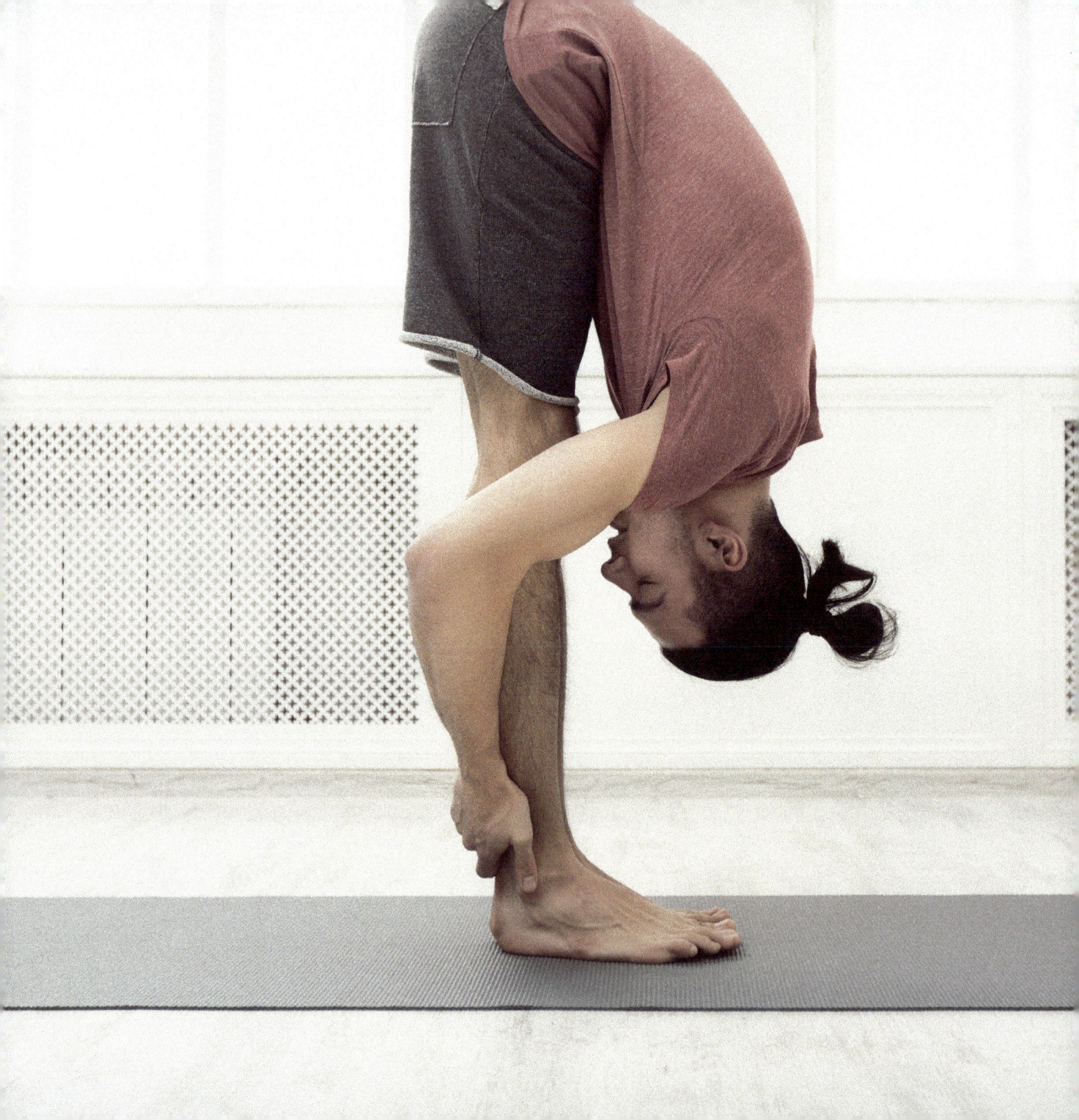

UTTANASANA - ACTIVE FORWARD FOLD / FORWARD BENDING POSE

OFF the Mat:

- Slows the heart rate and calms the mind, as the front body is protected and quieted
- Fosters positivity, a reversal of mild depression
- Boosts energy and can help in achieving more restful sleep

This pose has been likened to a human waterfall. It's a wonderful visualization. Your back body is the fresh, crystal clear water rushing down, and your front body is the quiet underneath it.

ON the Mat:

The most important thing to understand here is that this pose has nothing to do with touching your toes—read on:

KEY: Common mistake: making this about the reach of the arms and thus rounding the shoulders. This is all about the pelvis. After some hamstring and full body warmups, tilt your pelvis anteriorly such that you are lengthening the line between your belly button and public bone (sticking your booty out). That is what initiates this forward bend. Engaging the quads can help release the hamstrings.

- Once that is established, with newfound space between your groin and belly, your torso feels much freer to lower itself down

- Come down slowly and with a straight back, supported via the hands resting on the thighs
- Bend your knees if there is tension around your neck, back body or the backs of your legs
- To further modify, bring the floor up toward you via the use of blocks. Place a block (or textbook, anything works) outside of each foot and rest palms or tented fingertips upon them.
- There is an internal rotation of the thighs that works in tandem with the pelvic tilt (if you can't feel this, try squeezing a block between your thighs and pushing it backward...now remove the block and reestablish this sensation)
- If your body feels open enough to go further, reset the pelvic tilt, raising sitz bones to the sky and see if that gives you the additional space needed to remove any blocks and place tented fingers or palms flat on the ground (alternatively, you can hold the backs of the ankles)
- Wherever you have landed, let go of your neck, feeling the full weight of the head
- Stay engaged: This is an active forward bend, not a passive one

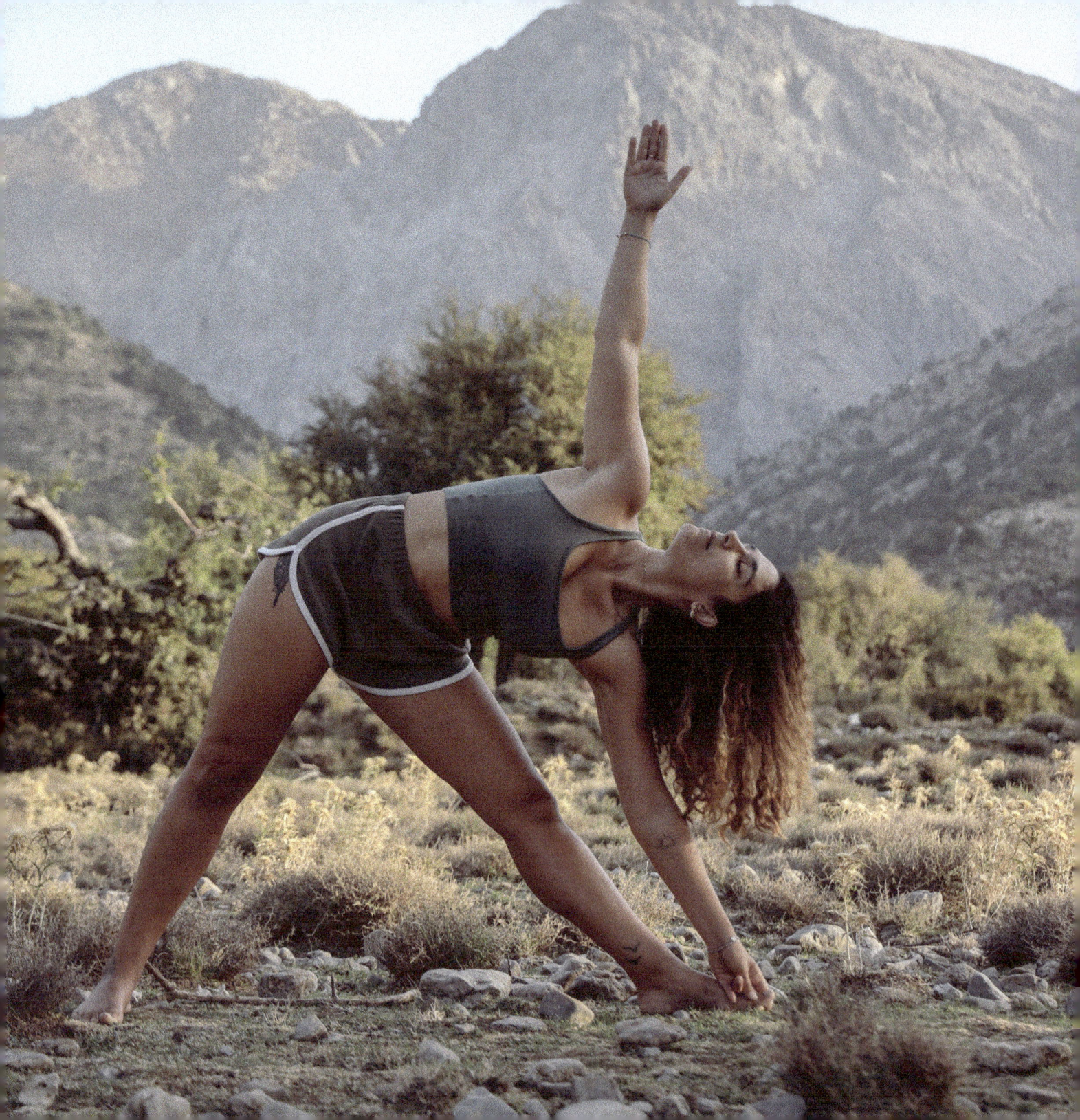

UTTHITA TRIKONASANA - EXTENDED TRIANGLE POSE

OFF the Mat:

While so many yogic postures have us contorted and crunched, this can feel like one of the most freeing, enjoyable poses ever. It's about opening and expanding the front and back bodies equally. We are balancing yin and yang, conservation/transformation, substance/energy, feminine/masculine, darkness/light, inner and outer parts of us.

ON the Mat:

A great set up pose for this one is Warrior II [see all three Warrior pose descriptions to come a bit further in this section]. It's the same feeling and positioning of the pelvis (front hip bones squared to the side you're facing, same leg placement).

- Standing with feet wide apart, about the distance of your outstretched arms (from wrist to wrist)
- The front leg is straightened, but not locked
- Energetically bring your back hip further back in space, leaving room in the front groin
- This allows you to literally hinge forward (note this specific phrasing: the torso stays completely engaged and in place as though frozen; the hinging motion at the hips descends it)
- Place your bottom hand wherever it can lie lightly. No dumping all your weight into the shin, ankle, or floor—activate your core to pull you slightly up so the hand rests gently
- Traditionally, the lower hand is placed on the front shin, ankle or, if flexibility allows, the ground behind the front foot (a block here can be helpful). Neither is better; do what works for your body in this particular moment.
- The top arm is raised straight above, reaching for the skies
- The arms are stacked: top wrist to top shoulder, directly overtop vertical collarbones, bottom shoulder to bottom wrist
- Though this pose is not a 'twist' in the traditional sense, there is a slight twisting of the torso; the top ribs are encouraged up and back, the bottom ribs roll slightly forward such that they stack
- Abdominals are engaged
- The gaze is upward toward the top hand (if stability and cervical spine health allow)
- Curl your tailbone in and under
- Breathe…and smile
- Switch sides

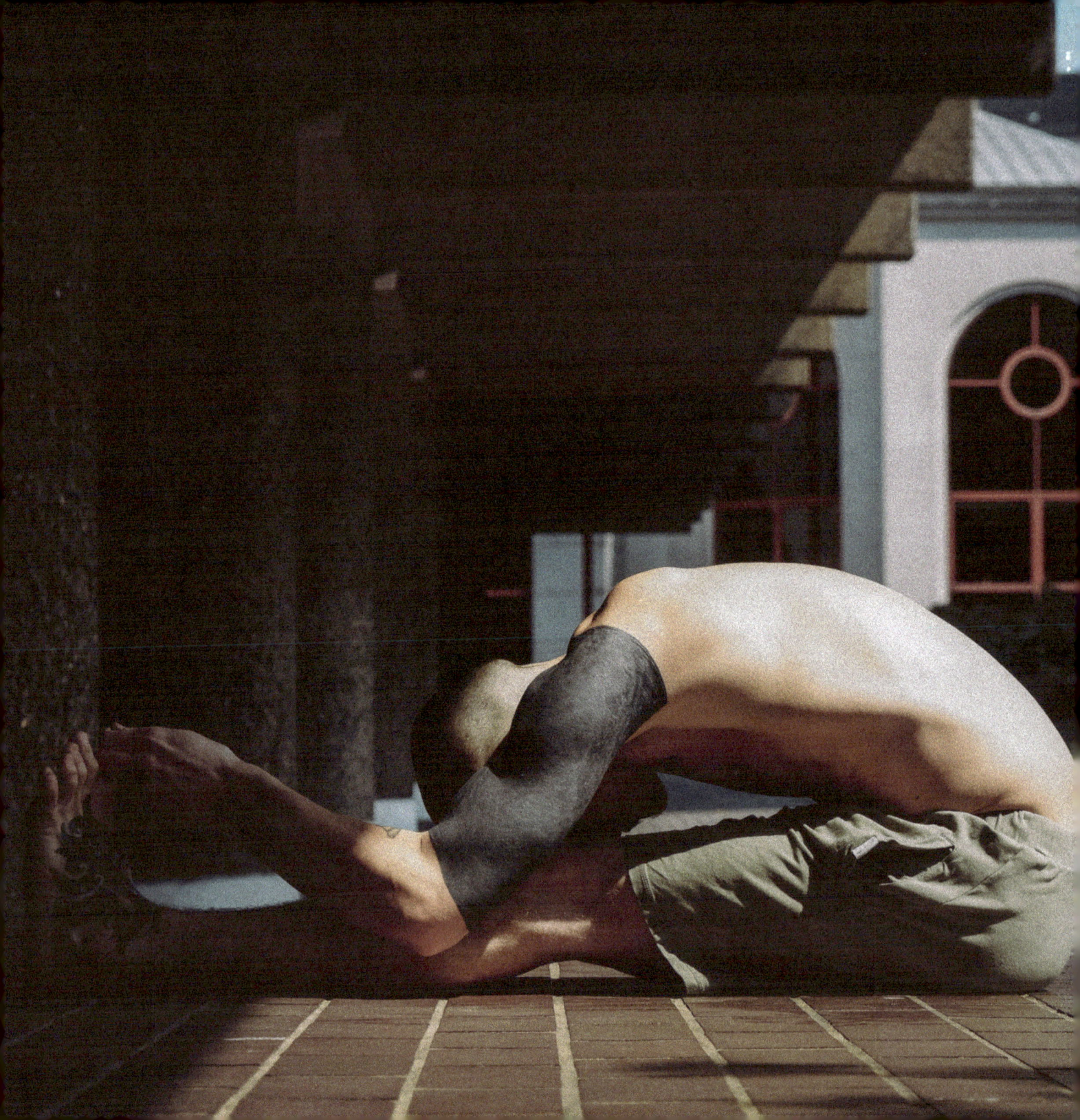

PASCHIMOTTANASANA - SEATED FORWARD BEND POSE

OFF the Mat:

* Paschimottanasana = "west-intense stretch"
(In yoga, the west is the entire back body)

- The back body is also seen as the past; in this and other forward folds we can release the past and the tensions that lay there
- Tension in the buttocks, backs of the legs and soles of the feet is often responsible for lower back compression and pain. Here, we focus on grounding and opening this area, often relieving chronic pain.
- Forward bends bring the mind inward, helping support calm introspection, preparing us for meditation

ON the Mat:

* Note: This pose is essentially Uttanasana (Standing Forward Bend), transposed

- Sit upright on the ground, legs outstretched in front, knees facing up and legs/feet parallel
- Pull the flesh out from under each sitting bone
- Energetically rotate your thighs internally—quadriceps moving in and pressing down while your toes stay pointing upward
- As with all forward folds, it's a bend that originates in the hip joint, not at the waist (remember this is a ball-in-socket joint, it has the potential for all kinds of mobility)
- Keep a gentle lift to the sternum and keep the torso long as you shift forward
- Sense that you are sending your sitz bones straight out behind you as your torso moves down (or, picture an anterior tilt of the pelvis, lengthening the area between your belly and groin)
- Go slow. Take your time by taking a few slow and deep breaths at your 'edge'. On the next breath, see if the body has opened a degree further. If so, go there, and stay for another few breaths. Long holds with calm, rhythmic breath is the key to safely opening the body.
- Many will bend at the knees to accommodate tight hamstrings. I find this negates the primary purpose of the pose, which is to intensely stretch the backs of the legs. Instead, keep your thighs and calves glued to the ground. Grab a strap and loop it behind the soles of the feet or just let your hands fall gently wherever they do if the feet aren't accessible.
- If flexibility allows without rounding the spine, hold the outsides of the feet, hold the big toes with your first two fingers and thumbs or (deeper still) grab hold of one wrist with the other hand, behind the soles of the feet with elbows out. In either hand position, the feet stay dorsiflexed with an emphasis on outer edges pulling back toward you.
- Keep shoulder blades coming together on the back
- The traditional pose is laying your forehead to your shins. Of course, this need not be where you go, today, five years from now, or ever!
- If your head happens to be close to your legs already, prevent forcing the neck down by placing a folded blanket or cushion between your head and your shins
- Breathe

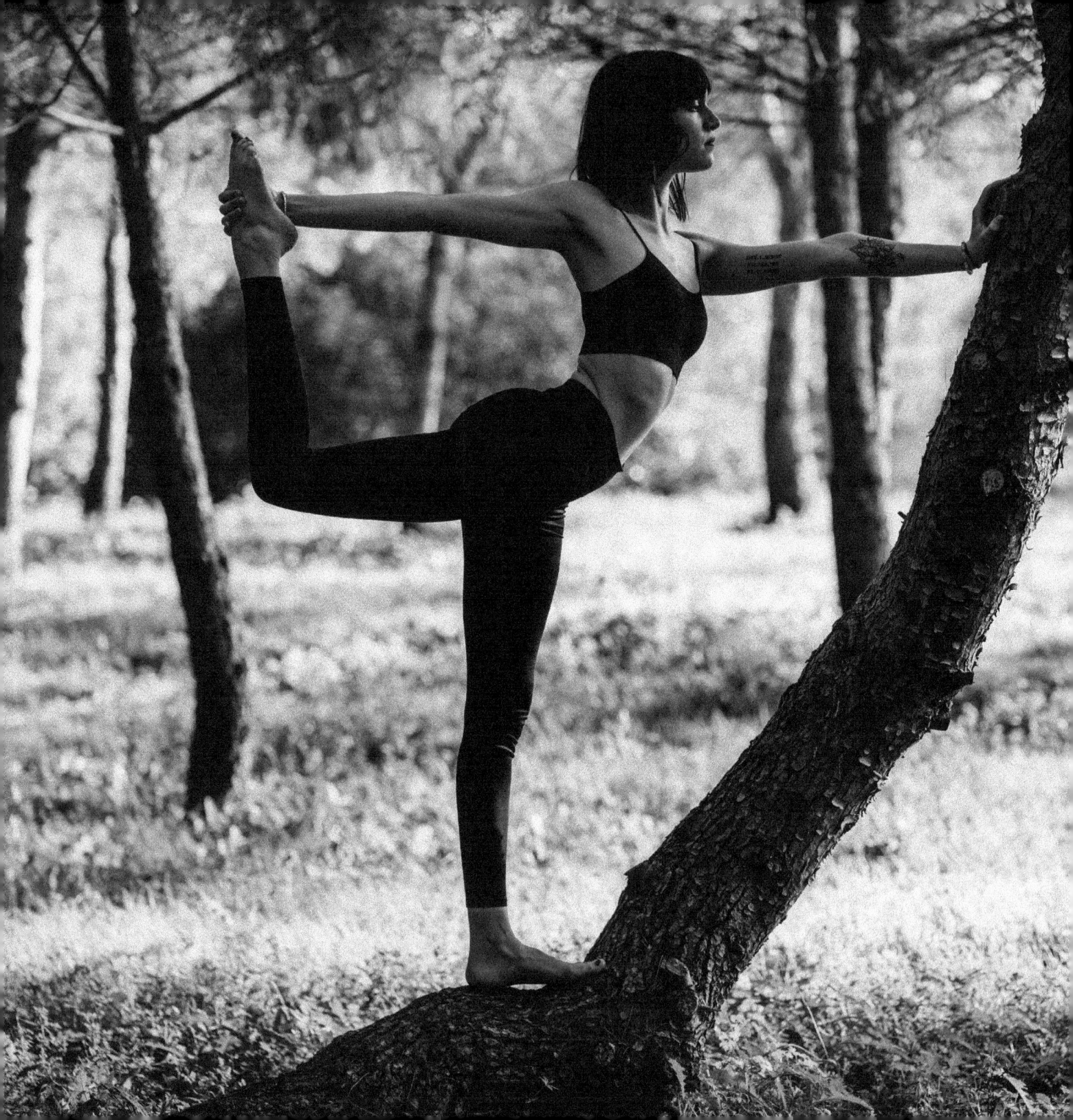

NATARAJASANA - LORD OF THE DANCE POSE / KING DANCER POSE

OFF the Mat:

- As a strong backbend, this pose opens the front body and, with it, various chakras—helping you regain a sense of abundance, well-being, self-esteem, and inner calm
- As a balancing posture, we also practice rooting firmly, finding ease and stability despite any gusts that attempt to shake us

Nataraja refers to the Hindu God Shiva who is a master of two opposing dances: one fierce and 'violent' (mostly in a good way, destroying mistaken beliefs that limit us) and the other tender, soft and loving. The pose calls us to reflect upon all the ways we can tap into both aspects of this graceful dance.

ON the Mat:

The most common mistake I see in this pose is opening the hip of the lifted leg in order to raise the foot higher. This is not meant to be a hip opener. To keep the integrity of this pose, rather, keep your hips in line with one another, both facing the floor/earth. This will also reposition your torso into alignment.

KEY: Make sure your hand holds the inner aspect of your foot versus the outer—the latter tends to pull that hip open, which we are trying to avoid

Another common mistake is moving the torso down low towards the floor. While there will be a subtle movement downward, do your best to keep upright as much as possible.

- Hips and shoulders should all be in line with one another, facing forward and somewhat downward
- Keeping all of the alignment principles just described, the raised foot will likely not rise as high... nobody ever won any yoga points for height. Always, always, alignment before ego
- Gaze/drishti is soft and to the horizon, keeping the chin slightly tucked
- Gently kick your foot into your hand, as though aiming for the wall or space behind you. Bring that same (holding) shoulder forward again if it strayed. We want the collarbones in one horizontal line in front of you, unslanted and untilted
- Avoid locking the knee of the standing leg. If it's suddenly harder and your muscles start shaking, you're in the right place.
- Lift the free arm straight-ish, bicep toward your ear, shoulder relaxed
- Breathe
- Switch sides

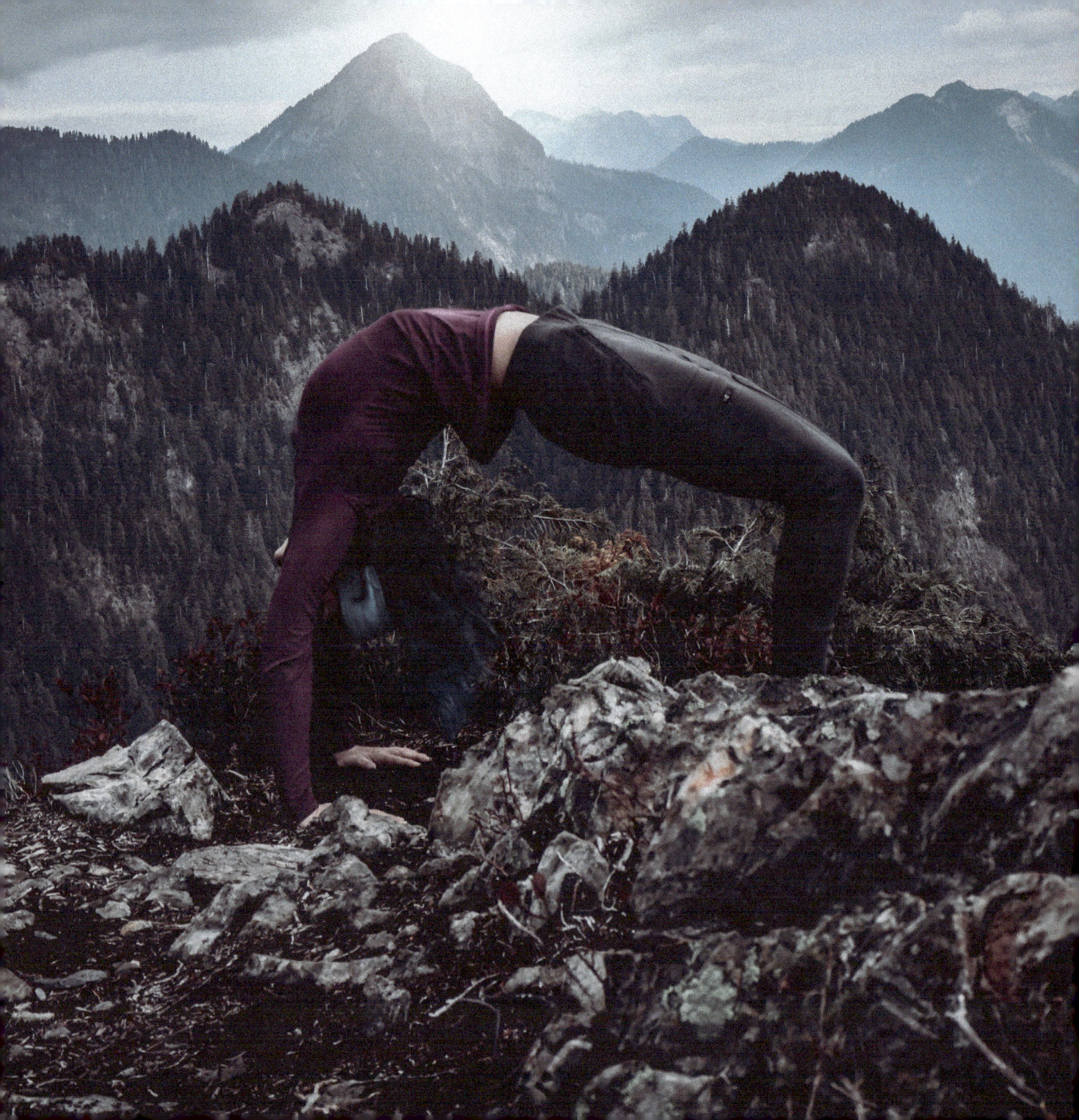

URDHVA DHANURASANA - WHEEL / UPWARD FACING BOW POSE

OFF the Mat:

- Known as "The Mother of all Backbends"
- Bolsters our ability to tolerate stress via direct action on the adrenal glands
- Strengthens determination and will power

ON the Mat:

This is a very deep posture and requires proper warming up. Warm the quads and hip flexors (low lunges, Hero's pose, King Arthur's pose), the spine (Bow pose, Bridge, Cobra) and shoulders (Eagle arms, Cow-faced arms). If your body isn't quite ready for Wheel Pose, practice Setu Bandhasana (Bridge Pose), which holds many of the same alignment and energetic principles.

- Lay down on your back and bend your knees so the feet are flat on the mat
- Feet are hip distanced and near parallel
- Move the buttocks closer to the heels (they can be touching but don't need to be)
- Inwardly rotate the inner thighs (keeping your knees from moving laterally) while pressing your big toes into the floor
- Bring your hands behind your shoulders, palms flat on the floor, fingers pointing toward feet
- Begin by pressing the lower back into the floor. The front aspect of the hip bones pulls away from the thighs toward your head and the tailbone tucks under toward the feet. Lift the tailbone (and rest of the spine) up in this way until you can place the crown of your head on the floor. No need to rush or push all the way up.

KEY: Two very important points to getting this right:

1. Hug the elbows IN (externally rotating the upper arms), creating space between your ears and your shoulder blades. Keep this going throughout the entire pose.

2. Push firmly into the palms and, instead of bringing your heart directly up toward the ceiling, send the sternum diagonally backward in space—that is, towards the edge of where the ceiling meets the wall behind you, away from your heels. Put another way, we send the torso and head diagonally away from your feet (rather than up), which allows your head to come between your arms and above your wrists. A common mistake is to have the wrists way out behind the head.

- Straighten the arms, continue to push down into the inner heels and big toes
- You may want to walk the feet in at this point if it works best with your body structure
- Though contested, you can slightly engage the bottom fibres of the glutes to prevent hyperextension/compression of lumbar spine as well as to make sure your knees don't splay outward
- If your body is open enough and you want more, walk the feet in further and the hands back, bringing the two closer together. Or stay right where you are.
- Breathe

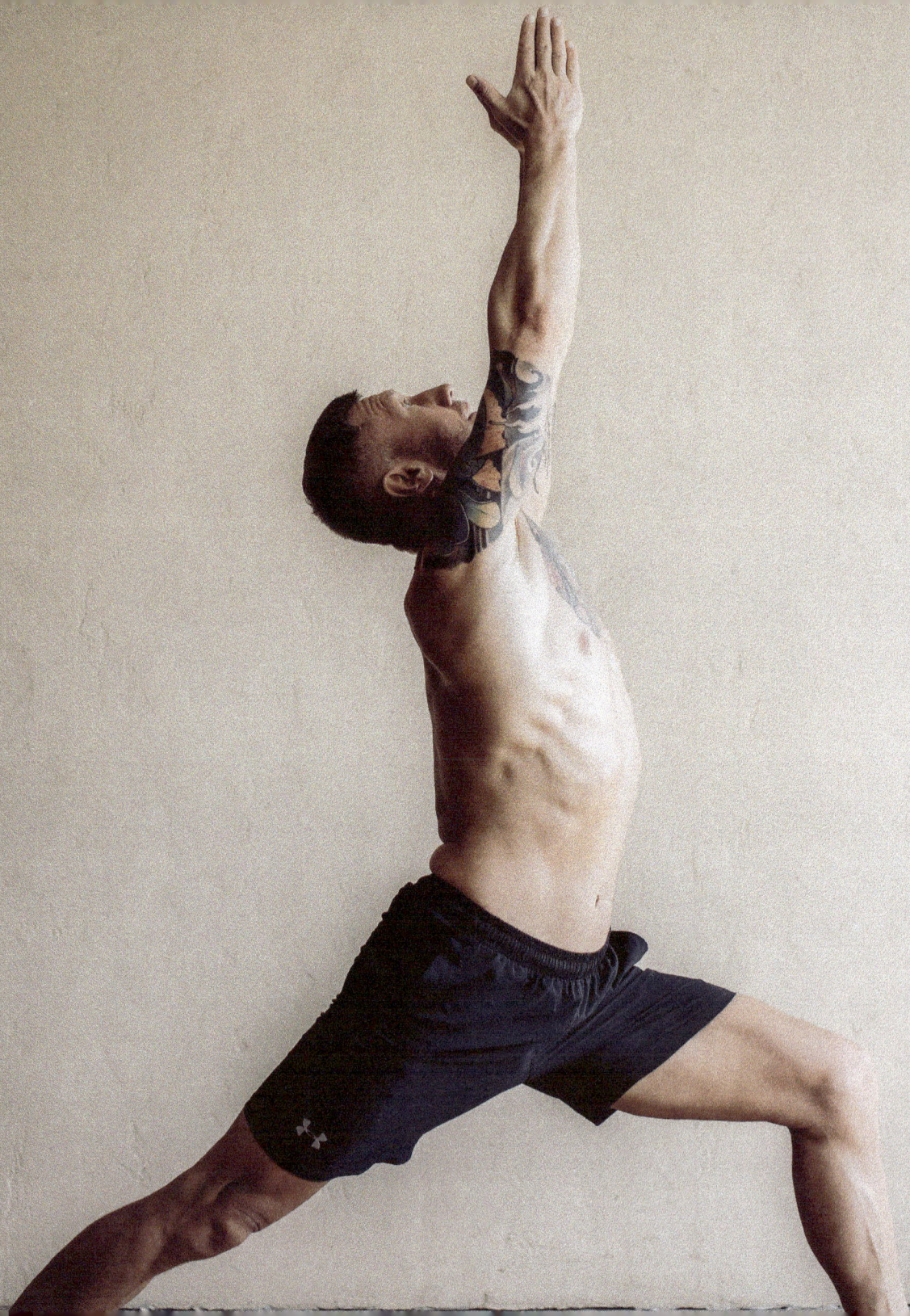

VIRABHADRASANA I - WARRIOR I POSE

OFF the Mat:

The warrior of yoga poses is an incarnation of Shiva (the destroyer). Caped in a tiger skin, this warrior has a thousand heads, a thousand eyes, a thousand feet and a thousand clubs. Instead of the outwardly violent image, it's truly about fierce, love-slaying ego. The energized arms are the warrior's sword.

And again, a balanced dualism reigns queen in this pose: lifting and grounded, forward and backward, stern and kind, strong and gentle, destructive and constructive.

- Can you hold all the physical components of this posture while keeping ease of mind?
- What must you let go of so that something new can be birthed?

ON the Mat:

- Wide stance running the length of your mat, feet about four to five feet apart
- Turn your front foot 90 degrees toward the front of the mat, and your back foot in about 25-40 degrees
- Gently rotate your torso (from hips to shoulders) in the same direction as your front foot
- Bend the front knee, ensuring it is stacked right above the ankle (it's common for the knee to come too far forward, watch for this and correct it)
- Lift your arms from the shoulder joint, extending active fingertips straight above you. Elbows are in toward your ears, palms inward, shoulders down and back. Hands can be together or apart
- Bring the fronts of both hip bones to point forward, in the same direction as your front foot and knee.

KEY: This is a challenge for most! The hip of the back foot will want to open outwardly, and the front hip will want to move forward. This pose requires consistent attention and rotational energy in the opposite direction: As far as your anatomy allows, pull the front hip back and the back hip forward. It can be helpful to place the wrists of open hands onto each front hip bone, fingers pointing forward (as though headlights), to get a better sense of the alignment happening here. Focus on lengthening the lower back (tailbone under, abdominals in and up) and slightly lifting the front hip toward the lower ribs. This will create the space you need, slowly, over time.

- Most of the weight of the torso is to fall on the inner aspect of the back buttock and the outer edge of the back foot. What the front thigh carries is minimal.
- Continue to bend into that front knee until the forward leg is at a right angle
- Straighten and lift the chest, bringing the lower ribs in
- Iyengar (alignment guru, master teacher) always emphasized maintaining the lift of the back knee, from heel to hamstring
- Face is relaxed, mind is passive
- Repeat on the other side

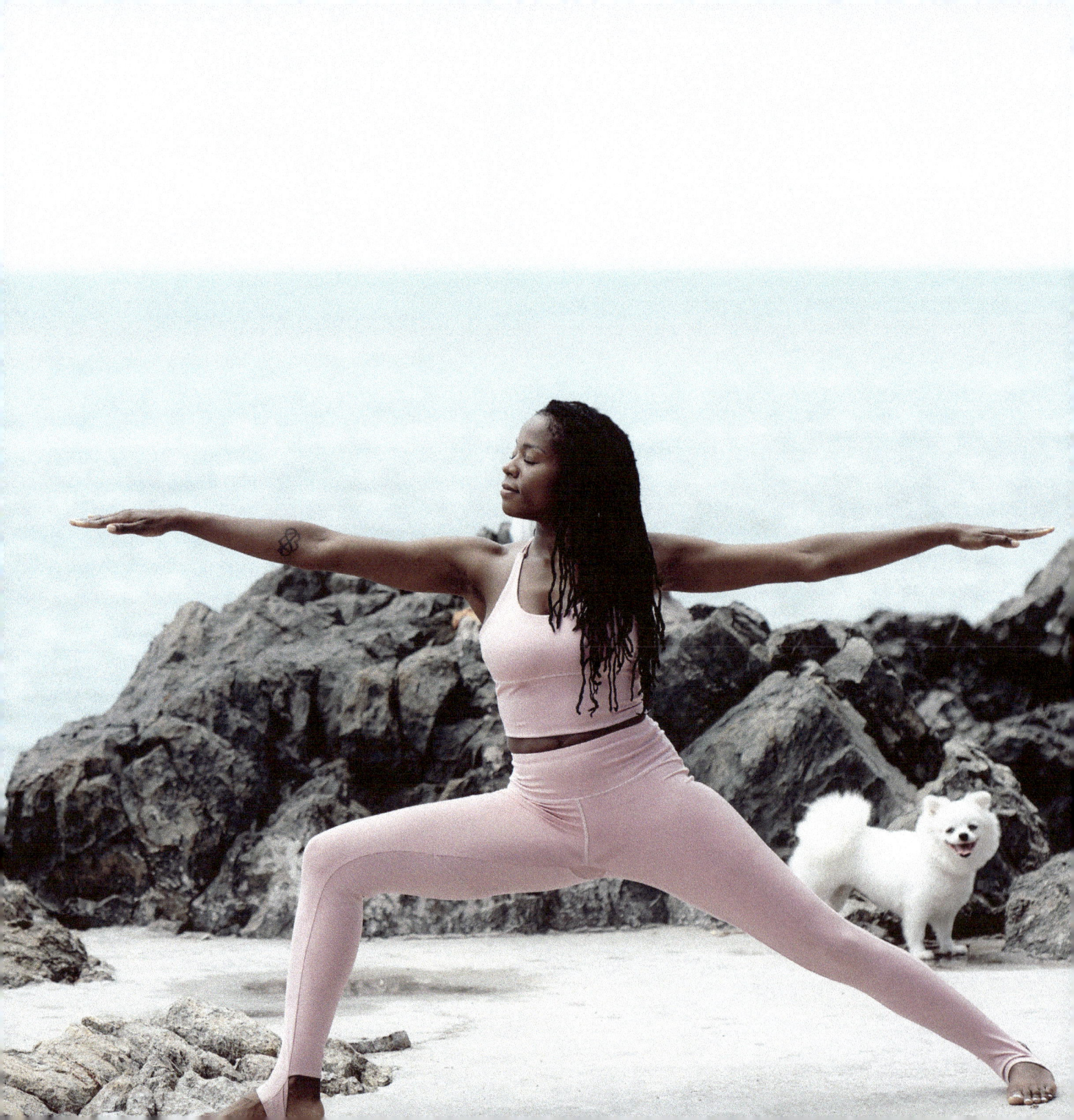

VIRABHADRASANA II - WARRIOR II POSE

OFF the Mat:

Embody the 'peaceful warrior'—this shifts our attention toward the centeredness that is prerequisite for any warrior in the throes of battle. Understanding where and how to place one's strength and at the same time one's mercy. In some circles of psychology, this is called the Wise Mind. Vira II, practiced regularly, helps strengthen this balanced mind within us.

Can you hold a soft, steady gaze out toward and beyond the fingers outstretched in front of you? Where are you looking, or headed? This attention will dictate where you go.

ON the Mat:

- Step your feet apart on the mat so they are parallel with the short edge of your mat. They should be about the same distance apart as in Vira I.
- The front foot is turned 90 degrees outwardly, towards the front of your mat. If you were to draw a straight line directly backward from your front heel, it would intersect the back foot at its arch.
- The knee of the front leg bends to form a 90 degree angle—work on opening the front thigh out in the same direction as the foot
- The back leg is straight and taut
- The weight of the upper body is evenly distributed below, on both the heel of the front foot and the 4th and 5th toes of the back foot (micro-shift your weight until you've struck a balance between them)
- Keep the hips open, turning them slightly away from the front leg
- The tailbone is down, the abdominals engaged
- Raise both arms to parallel with the floor—one straight out in front and one behind you
- Fingers are energized, not locked, head is turned forward and gaze is over the front fingers, looking beyond them (chin slightly in, face soft)

The most common mistake I see in this pose is leaning too far forward with the torso and the front arm. Remember, this pose is about holding centeredness above all. To ensure you are in proper alignment, check that your front armpit is directly atop your front hip.

- One of my favourite tricks to ensure strong but relaxed arms is to gently flip both palms skyward, kissing the shoulder blades together on the back and seeing where release is possible. After finding it, rotate only the palms back to face the earth, maintaining all of the shoulder and arm opening just established.
- Gain height by consciously lifting both sides of the torso
- When you're ready, switch sides

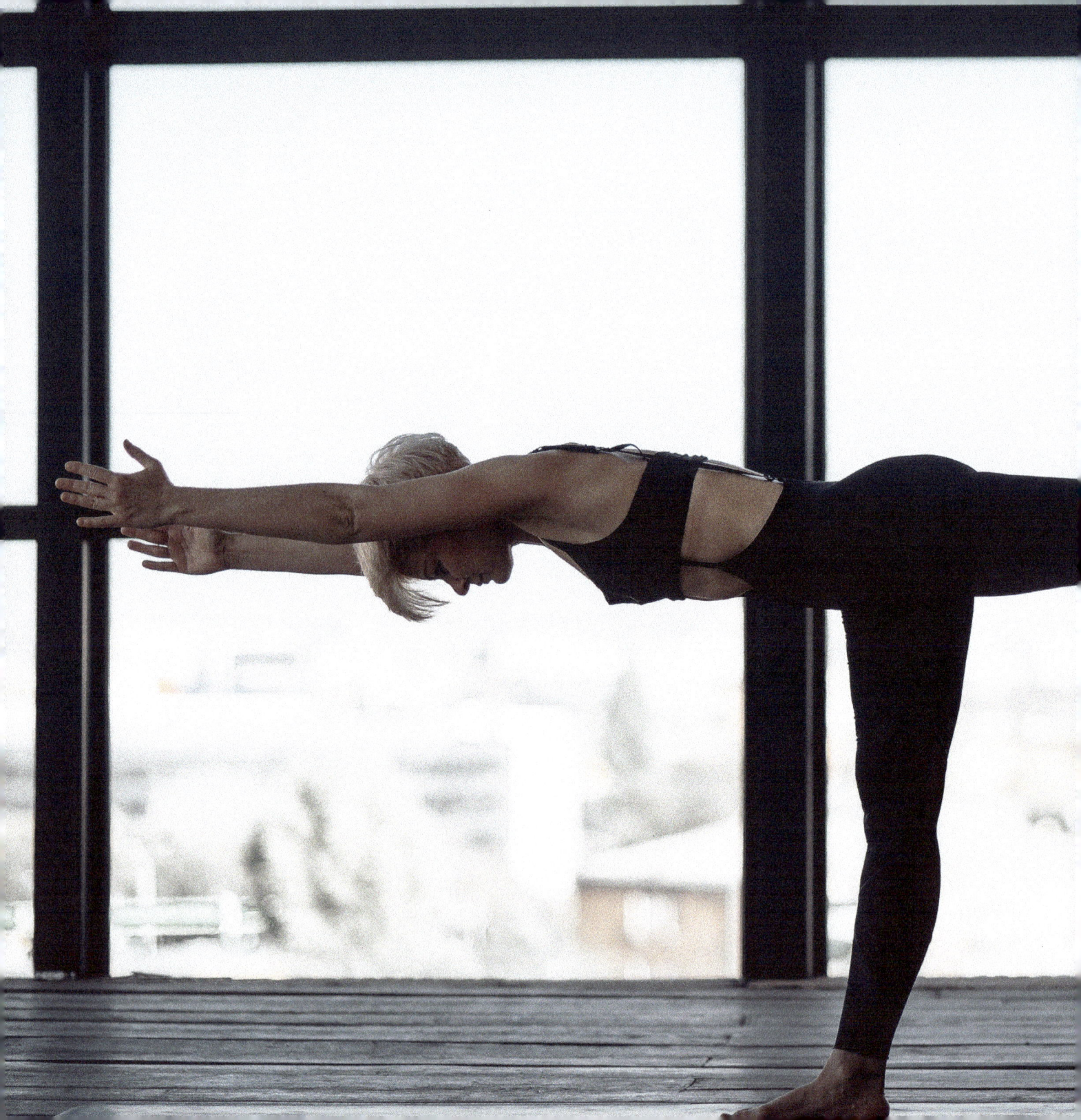

VIRABHADRASANA III - WARRIOR III POSE

OFF the Mat:

Here, again, is Shiva—cultivating love that is strong, wild, and untamed.

- Builds strong balance and proprioception
- Improves memory, focus and concentration
- Quiets the mind, calms anxiety and the nervous system

ON the Mat:

- Like so many postures, getting this pose 'right' anatomically is all about where the hips are in space. Use your proprioception (your awareness of your body in space) to get comfortable feeling the pelvis—its tilt and position on both sides.
- Start by standing tall, in Tadasana
- Shift weight into one leg, and consciously lift the other toward the wall behind you
- When lifting the back leg, the tendency is to tilt the hip out to the side and upward to falsely get more height. Instead, point the front of that hip down toward the ground until you feel both front hip bones are level and pointing to the earth beneath you.
- Shift a bit on your standing leg such that your weight is balanced on all four corners of the foot, strongly down into the big toe
- Bring the hip of the standing leg a bit backward in space to even out the pelvis and ensure the head of the thigh bone sits into its hip socket
- Once you have your balance, the standing leg is to be slowly straightened but not locked. The slight micro-bend makes this pose so much... stronger.
- Find a focused gaze (drishti) to help anchor you
- Save for the standing leg, attempt to have everything else (arms, torso, head, and neck) parallel to the floor
- The traditional pose is to have the arms out in front, in line with the ears, either shoulder width apart (as seen here) or in prayer toward the wall in front of you. Bring your shoulders gently backward ('down' the body) and away from your ears to prevent shrugging.
- It can be very helpful to pull both thighs energetically toward one another (imagine squeezing a block between them)
- The neck is in line with the rest of the spine, gaze upon the toes or just ahead of you
- Abdominals engaged, belly button in and up
- Extend equally in opposing directions with the back leg backward and upper body forward
- The hands and feet are engaged as well, energy in both
- Maintain a smooth, steady breath
- Use a wall or a chair in front of you if you find your balance isn't yet sufficiently developed. It will be, just keep practicing.
- Reset to neutral, then repeat on the other side

* A modification of this arm position is airplane pose, where the arms point backward along the body.

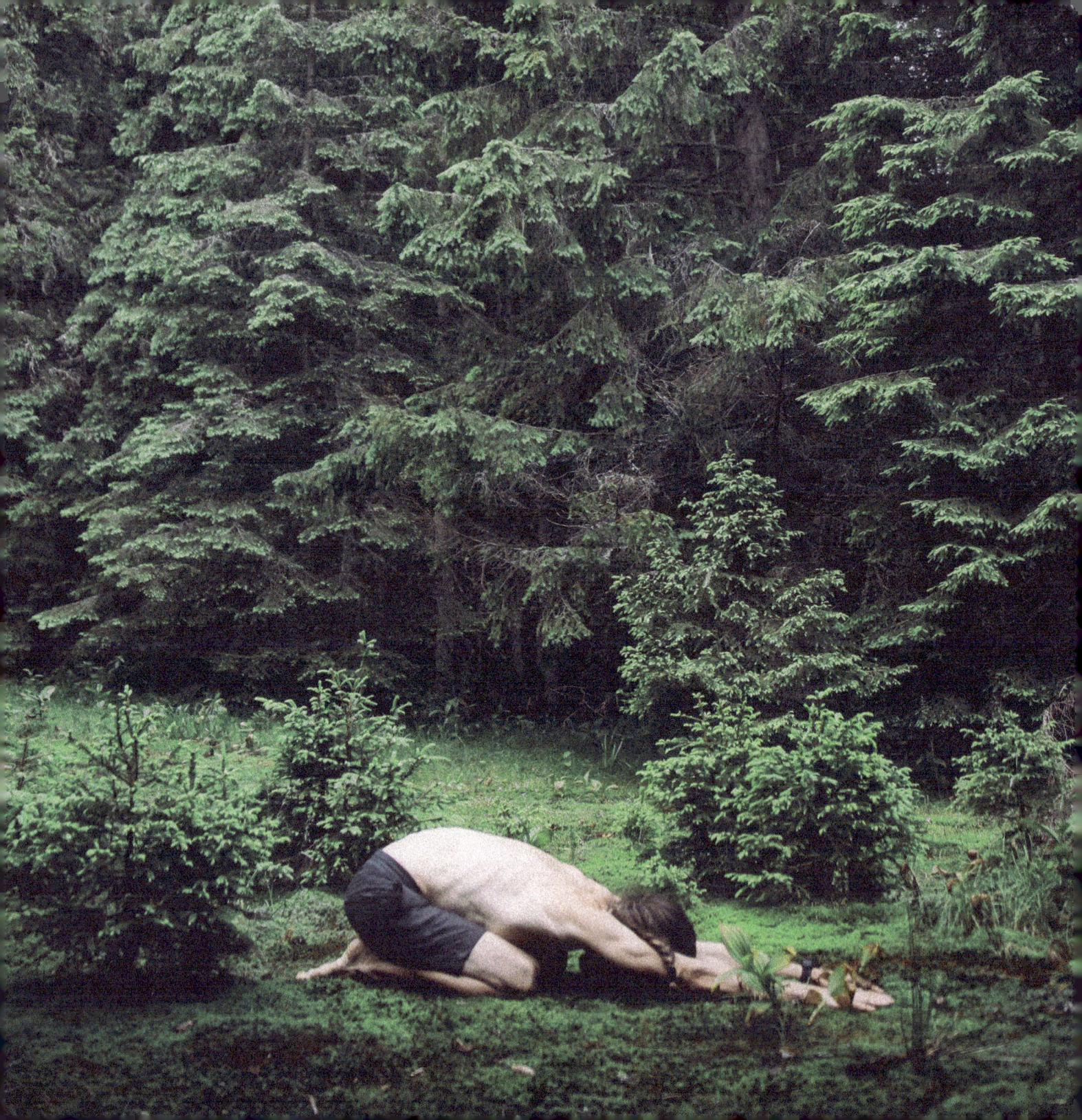

BALASANA - CHILD'S POSE

OFF the Mat:

While Balasana can be an opportunity to take rest during a challenging sequence, it is also an opportunity to go much deeper in our body and breath awareness:

- Here, the ribcage and abdomen are compressed, making our usual breathing patterns difficult. As with all postures, we work with the pose rather than against it—adjusting our breath as well as our bodies such that the inhale and exhale can rhythmically continue, despite the constriction. With awareness, we learn to breathe into the open areas. Here, we send breath behind the heart, filling the back of the lungs and allowing the sides of the ribcage to open outwardly. A focused breath practice (like Ujjayi/Victorious Breath) can be very helpful here.

- Allows introspection and protected vulnerability while releasing the past
- Supports yin building (sorely lacking in our busy lives)
- Massages and tones the digestive organs
- Calms the mind

ON the Mat:

- Sit back on your heels, toes together and untucked such that the tops of your feet lay on the mat
- Bring the bent knees out laterally to about hip width
- On an exhale, hinge at the hips to bend the torso forward (rather than curving the spine)
- Extend the arms out in front of you, and rest your hands, torso and forehead softly down on the earth beneath them. You may use blocks, stacked fists or hands underneath the forehead, if either helps make this accessible.
- Resist the urge to lift your hips in order to reach your hands further forward. Always, always, integrity in the pose. Hips stay well back, energetically shooting the tailbone out behind you. If your body doesn't yet allow the hips to stay rooted on the heels, place a bolster or rolled up towel between them.
- Widen your sitz bones to allow more of an opening in the sacrum
- Ensure there is a healthy space between the back of your neck and the base of your skull by imagining that continuous line of the spine, from tailbone to the very top of the neck
- As you breathe and really enter the pose, you may, in time, gain the depth to shift your torso and head forward on the ground (while maintaining rested hips on heels)

* One variation of this is having the arms and hands behind you, palms up. Here the front shoulders can be released onto the floor by relaxing and opening the space between the shoulder blades.

* Another variation is with knees together, resting the torso on the tops of the thighs.

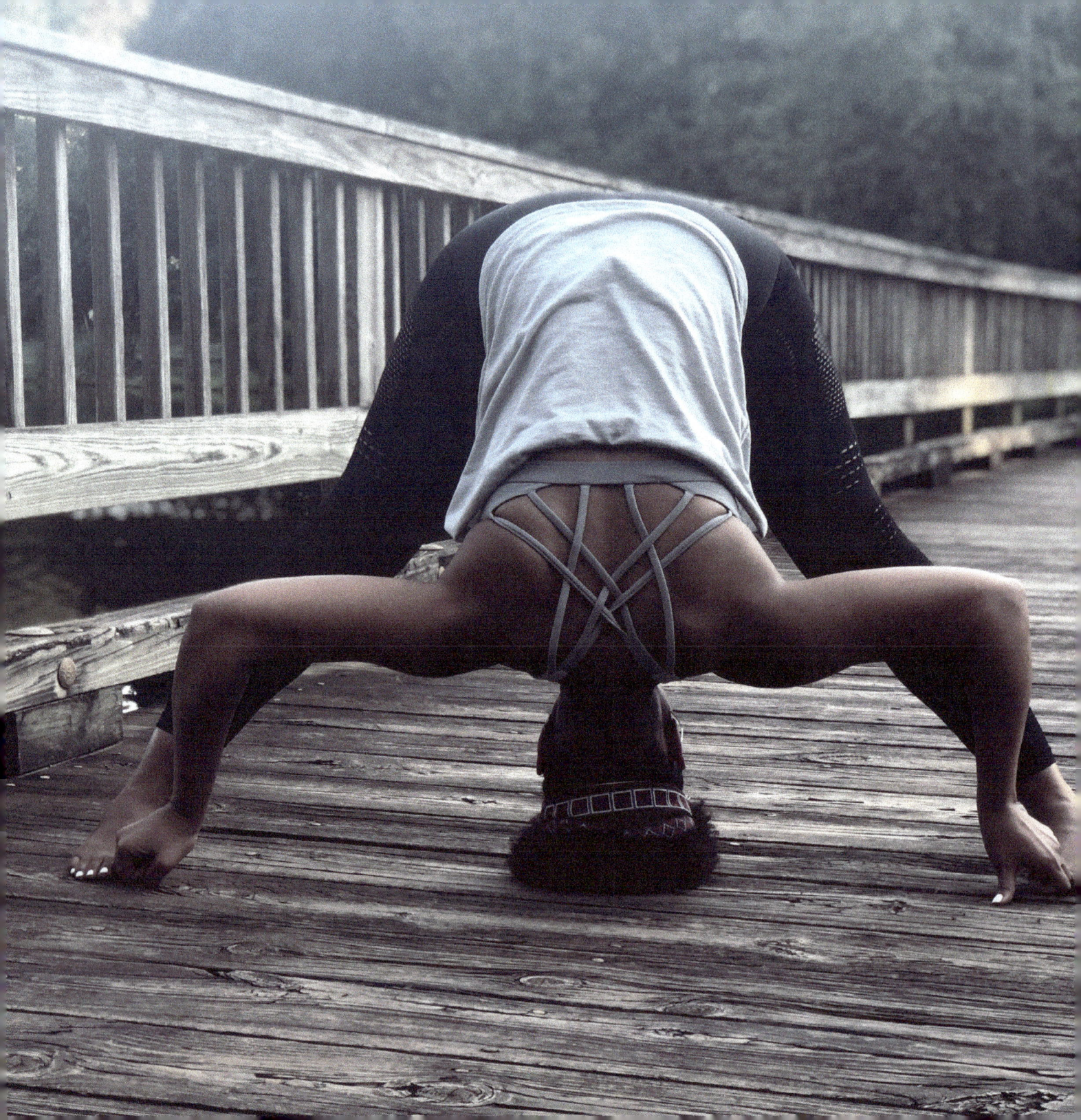

PRASARITA PADOTTANASANA - WIDE-LEGGED STANDING FORWARD BEND

OFF the Mat:

- According to Iyengar, this pose cools down the brain and body and calms the practitioner
- Lowers blood pressure
- Soothes migraines, tension headaches and fatigue
- Head to Earth: humbles the mind/ego

ON the Mat:

- Come to the base pose by either jumping or stepping your feet out to about 4 meters apart, lengthwise on the mat (adjust according to your leg length and flexibility)
- Feet parallel to the short edges of your mat (sometimes the toes are pointed very slightly inward). Lateral edges of the feet should be firmly planted.
- Avoid rounding the back to enable reaching the floor; we hinge at the front hip creases, keeping the spine concave, looking forward, rather than rounding down
- Start with your hands at the hips. Now hinge forward, and as you lower the upper body, bring hands flat on the floor under the shoulders.
- With continued concavity in the back, walk your hands back in line with your feet if this works in your body
- Two common arm options here: Either root the fingerpads to the earth and bend the elbows backward, or reach hands to feet and hold the big toes with your peace fingers and thumbs (as shown here).
- In either option, guide the sternum 'forward' through

the legs and towards the wall/space behind you
- If it's possible to do so without rounding the back or neck, bring the crown of the head gently between your hands. If your low back or any injury prevents getting to this depth safely, use a bolster / folded blanket / cushion or yoga block to rest the top of the head.
- Make sure not to twist your head once it is touching the ground or prop
- Keep the torso long
- Activate the backs of the legs and push the feet and hands firmly into the mat to take any pressure off of the head and neck
- Like with other forward bends, think of energetically lengthening the backs of the thighs by pointing your sitz bones further up towards the sky or ceiling
- Un-shrug your shoulders away from your ears and widen the space between the shoulder blades
- Adjust the distance between the feet as your body requires—if the head seems to reach the floor too easily, shorten your stance. If, instead, it feels much too far away, widen your stance.
- Breathe

* Many variations to this pose exist. Iyengar taught versions A through D; both of the options above, as well as having hands on the hips with the head off the floor, and having the hands interlaced behind and away from the body.

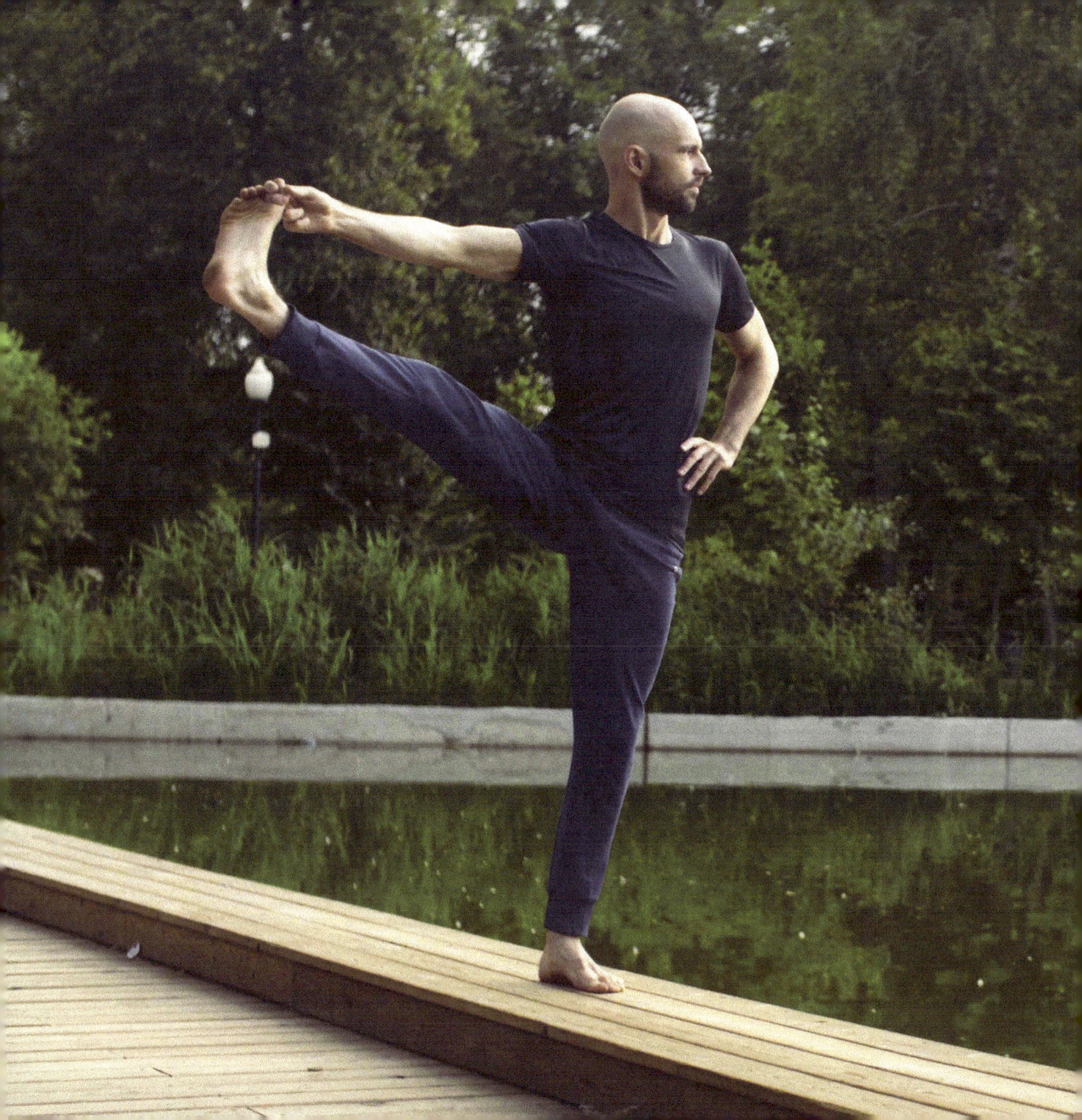

UTTHITA HASTA PADANGUSTHASANA - EXTENDED HAND TO TOE POSE

OFF the Mat:

Yoga is a constant push/pull. It's about shooting energy away and simultaneously toward. There are always opposing forces at play that require awareness and attention. This pose embodies all these dualities and allows us, when practicing honestly, to be truly steady and at ease.

- Improves focus, concentration and balance
- Builds a strong connection to the breath

ON the Mat:

If your hamstrings are tight enough that you are tucking the pelvis, rounding the spine, shrugging the shoulders, and/or grimacing at every step, look up online tutorials or ask a local instructor to help you work with blocks and straps to allow you to slowly open into the asana while keeping alignment intact.

- Stand steadily using a drishti straight across from you. Hands on your waist. Bring the full weight of the body onto one leg.
- Slowly lift the other leg straight out in front of you
- Bend the knee of your lifted leg into your side body, arm on the inside, as in Happy Baby pose. You can bring your two peace fingers to wrap around the lifted big toe. Modify by holding your shin if you cannot reach the toes or use a strap. You may stay here.

- Strengthen the abdominals and drive the standing leg energetically down through the earth to help steady and root you
- With toe or shin grasped, slowly extend the leg out in front (unbend the knee) while keeping the pelvis level. The heel pushes out and forward while the same hip moves back in toward its socket. Keep it bent or use a strap if it cannot extend all the way without losing alignment integrity. No matter your variation, keep the knee pointing to the sky, rather than out to the side.
- Only lift the leg insofar as you can keep the pelvis level. If the hip of the lifted leg begins rising up higher than the other, you've gone too far
- The shoulders relax down away from the ears, and are in line with one another. Take care to avoid jutting that shoulder forward but instead bring it back into its socket. You may stay here.
- If you are going further, hinge at the hips and bring your nose towards your lifted shin and vice versa. Only if you can keep breathing!
- To reach the pose as shown here: re-straighten the torso. If you have your balance, open the hip of the lifted leg by moving the hand/foot pair laterally away from your body. Transfer your gaze slowly in the opposite direction.
- Hold steady and breathe
- Switch sides

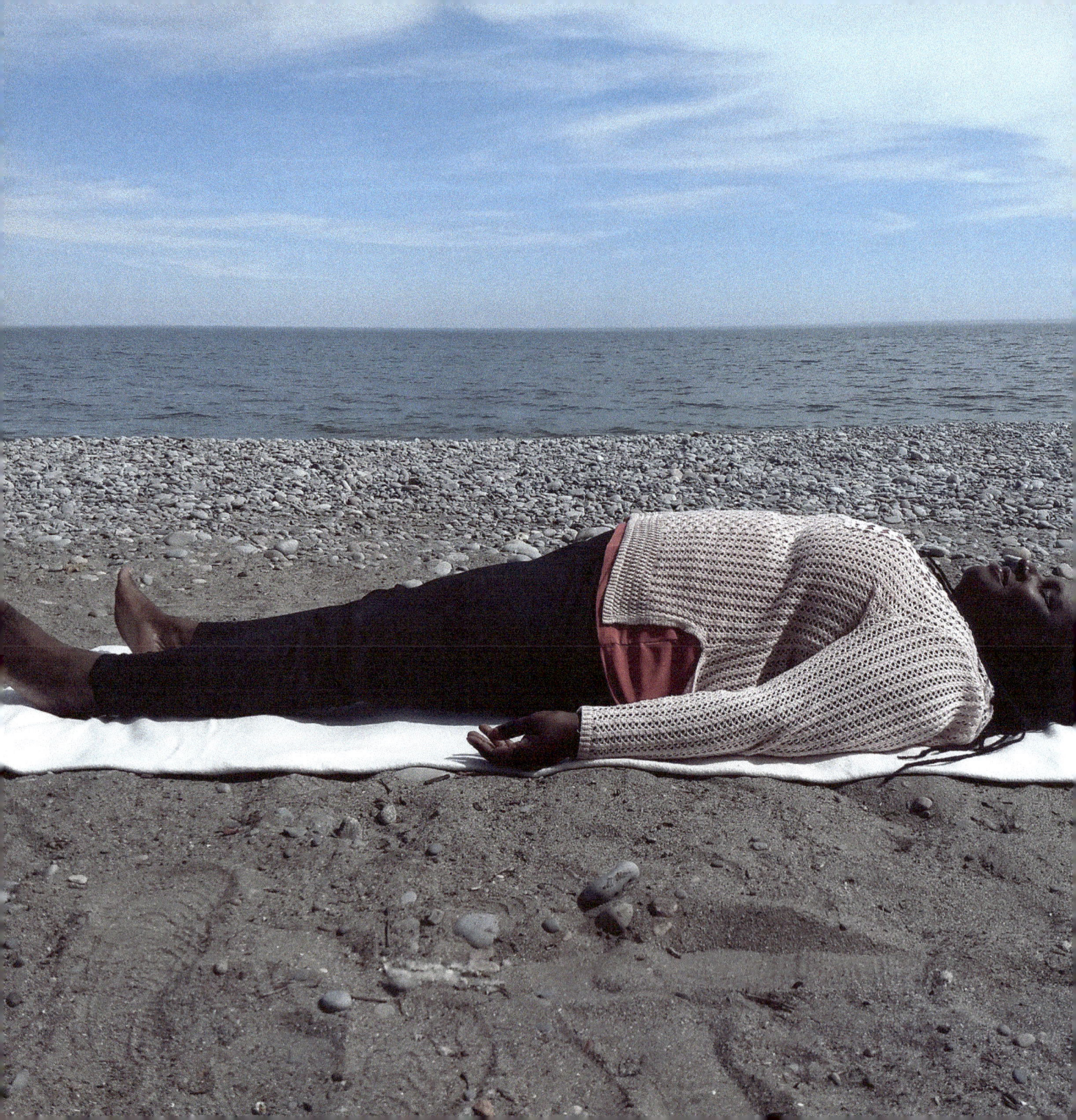

SAVASANA - CORPSE POSE

OFF the Mat:

You either love this pose, or you avoid this pose at all costs. You just don't have the time, or, you budget extra time to make sure this is unrushed. If you tend to skip it, I urge you—do not. Read on:

- Savasana is usually regarded as the most important pose of an asana practice; we unblock pranic energy (Qi / Life Force) as we move through all the other postures and then, in Savasana, all is integrated. The prior activity helps ease us into this pose's passivity.
- This is where we lie still. Where the doing is done. Here, all of the fruits of your practice come together. They swirl around as though in a singing bowl, gently mixing with equal parts catharsis, surrender and connection.
- It is a deeply restorative posture, allowing the nervous system a few moments of significant rest and a welcomed return to the parasympathetic state
- If your mind tends to race when in such non-doing states, it may be helpful to practice a simple visualization; a gentle body scan, being bathed in light, something to anchor your mind without overstimulating it
- The 'death' here allows for new beginnings—we come out of the pose rebirthed, renewed, with only the here and now upon us

ON the Mat:

- Lie on your mat or directly on the Earth with your legs long, about the width of the mat.
- Let your feet fall outward
- Eyes are gently closed
- Arms are at about a 45-degree angle away from your torso, hands and fingers open, palms up
- Shoulders are down and away from the ears
- Feel the weight of the head on the ground. Bring your chin down enough so that it is parallel to the ground rather than pointing up—this will lengthen the back of your neck.
- Slightly lift your hips and tuck the tailbone under and toward your heels. Now rest your hips gently back down.
- Notice any effort in the face and then soften: Release the tongue, relax the space between the eyebrows, unclench the teeth and jaws.
- Let go of everything: slowly scan your body from the tips of your toes to the crown of the head, letting go of every muscle, every energetic 'holding' along the way. By bringing the attention to each area, we push our surrender even further. The places we thought we were already letting go suddenly and completely fall even more deeply into the Earth.
- Let go of focused breath. Make this a conscious choice. Trust that your body will breathe you.
- Be still. Resist the urge to fix your clothes or hair, resist wiping sweat away or scratching an itch. After the initial adjustments of setting up the pose, be truly still. Stay present.
- Remain for at least 10-15 minutes. The benefits are revealed the longer you stay.

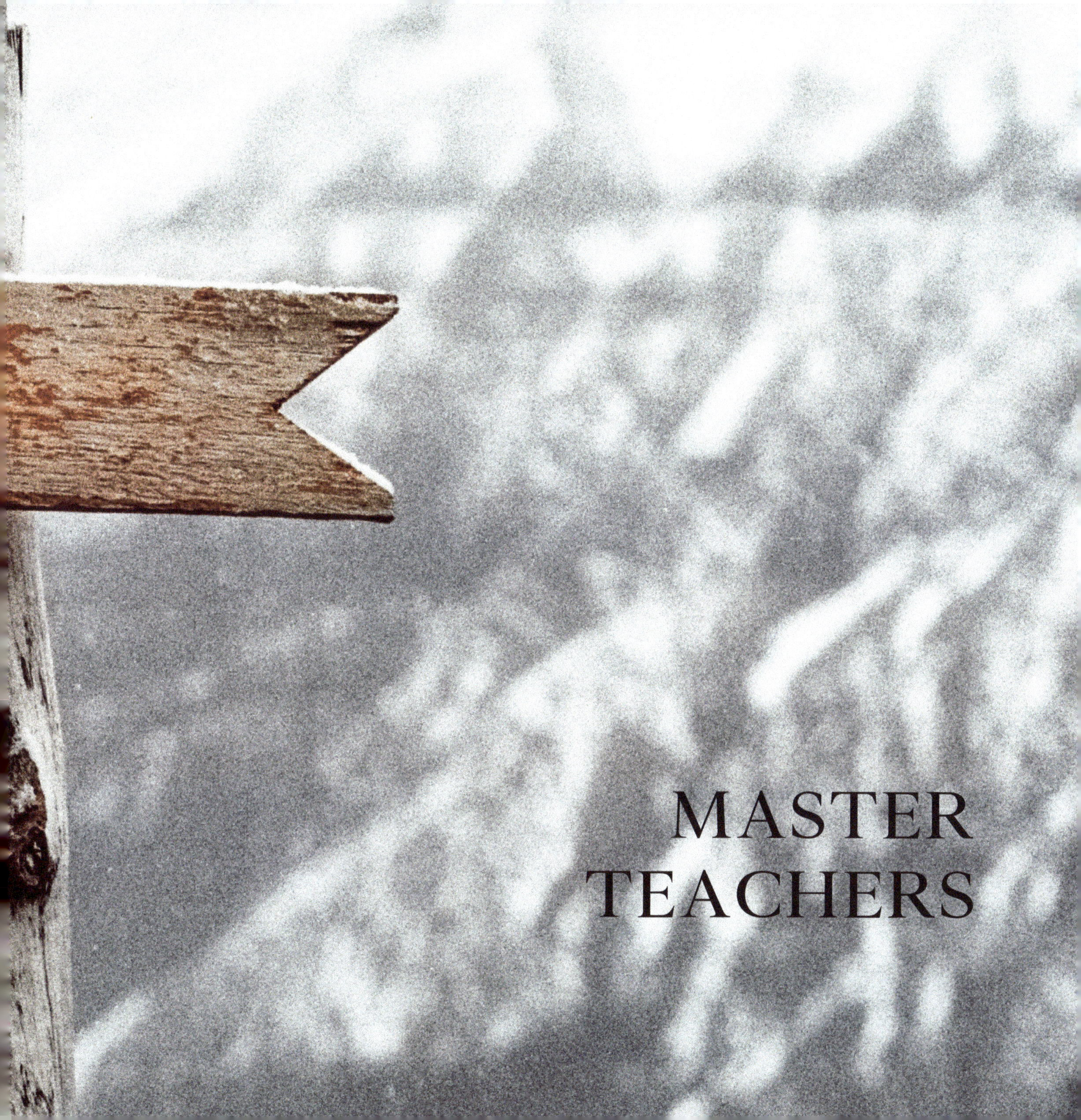

MASTER
TEACHERS

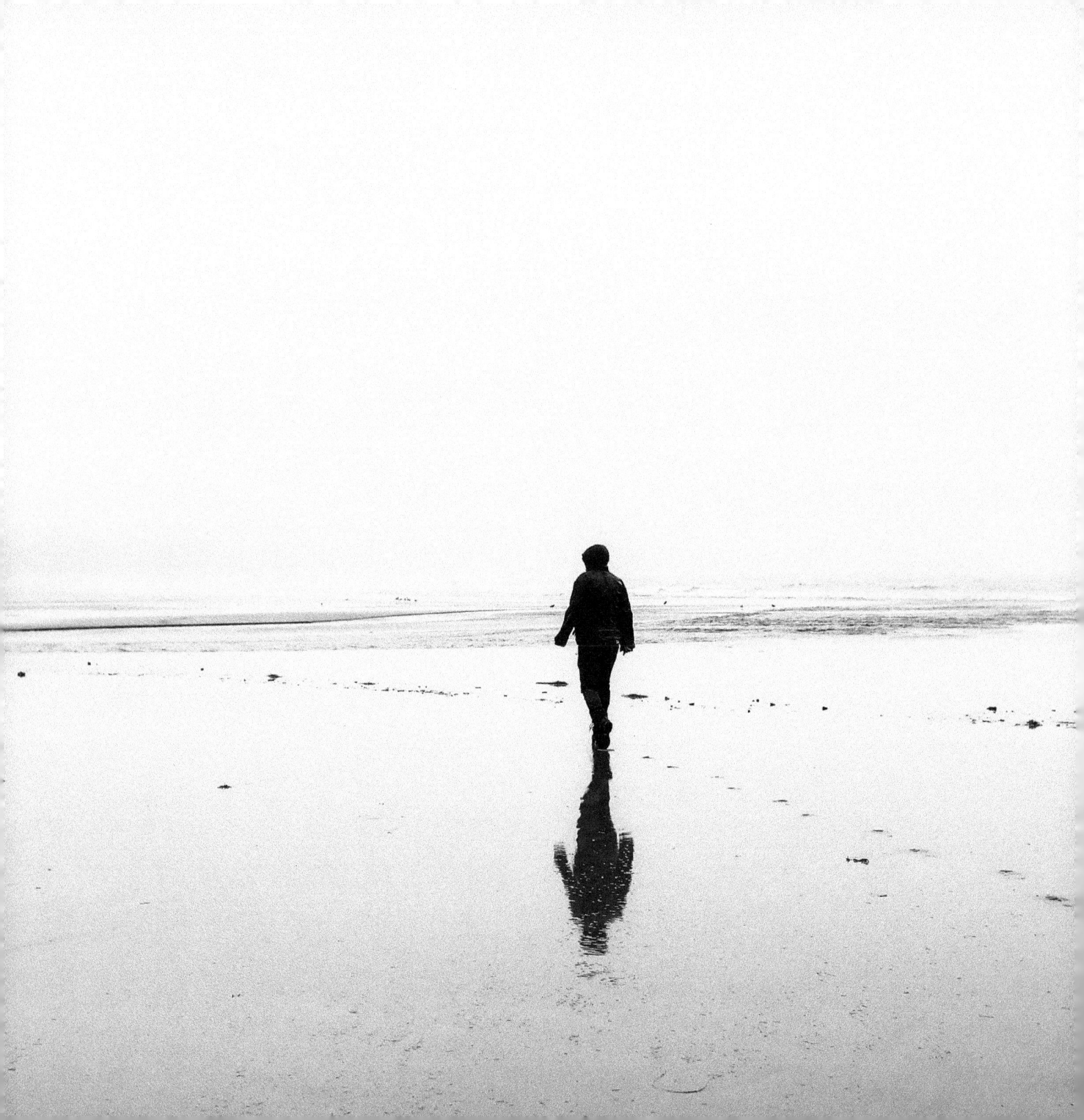

"The quieter you become,
the more you can hear."

-

RAM DASS

"I can't meditate," "I'm not good at meditation," "I have too many thoughts swimming around." I hear this from patients, family, and friends all the time.

Meditation Foundations: The idea that meditation equals making your mind blank while sitting upright in lotus posture is absolutely false.

Here's the rub:
The busy mind IS it.

It's the thing. It's why we're sitting in the first place. And it's the raw material we are working with. Without the busy mind or the mind that is anywhere-but-here, without the chatter and the noise and the overwhelming inputs from within and without, without the "interfering" emotions, there is no practice.

If you think you're failing at meditation but you're showing up to sit—you're winning! That's the exercise. You show up for Day one for whatever time you have. Five minutes? That qualifies. And then you show up for Day two. And Day three and four and you keep committing to trying. That's the practice.

The best part? When you think you are accomplishing nothing day after day, but you stay the course and sit anyway, the benefits creep up on you very quietly.

One day you're about to react "as usual" and, instead, you take a breath. You decide to choose a kinder action instead of an automatic, harsher reaction. You feel more the calm witness and less the tumultuous waters. You become who you want to be.

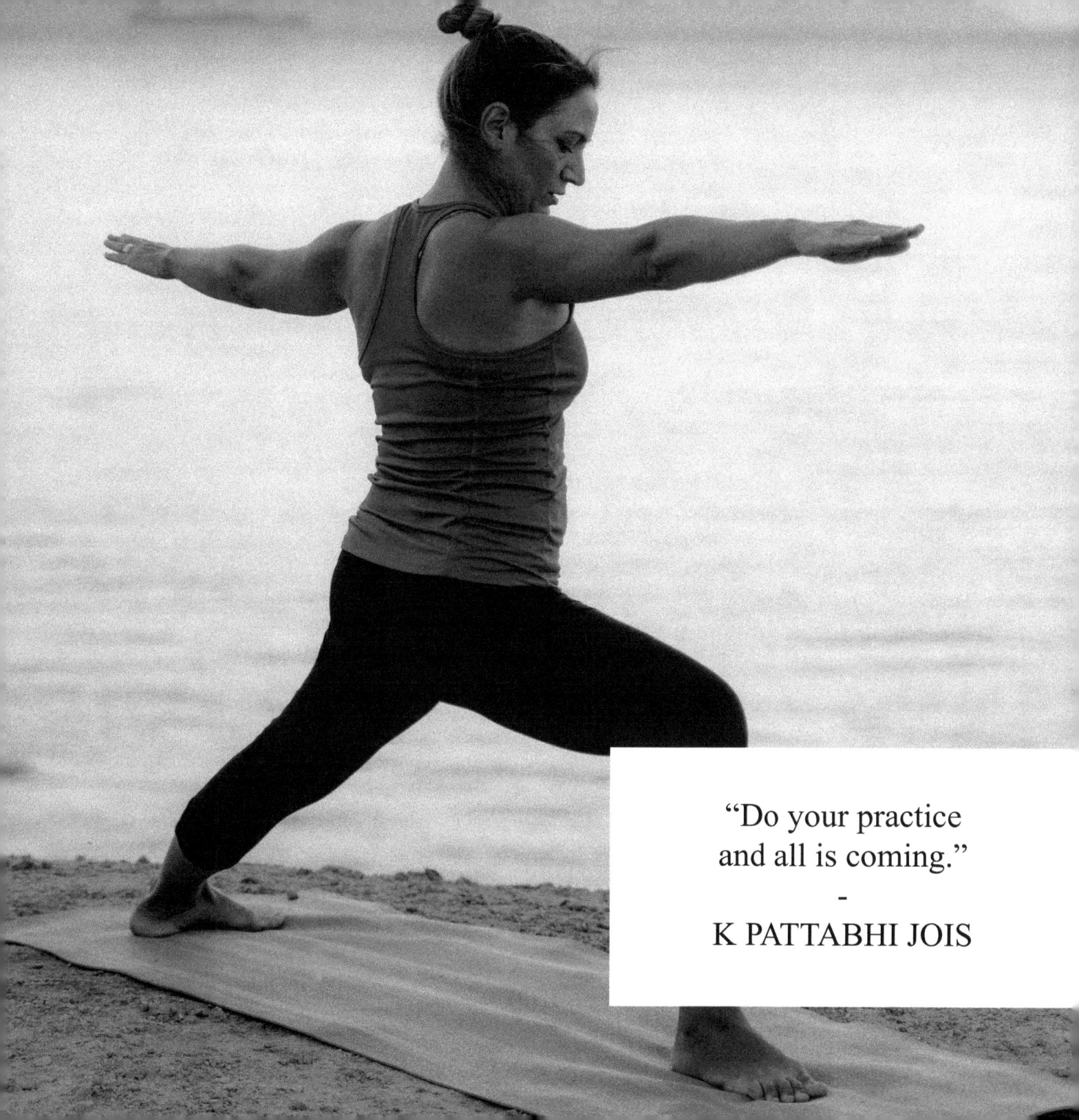

"Do your practice
and all is coming."
-
K PATTABHI JOIS

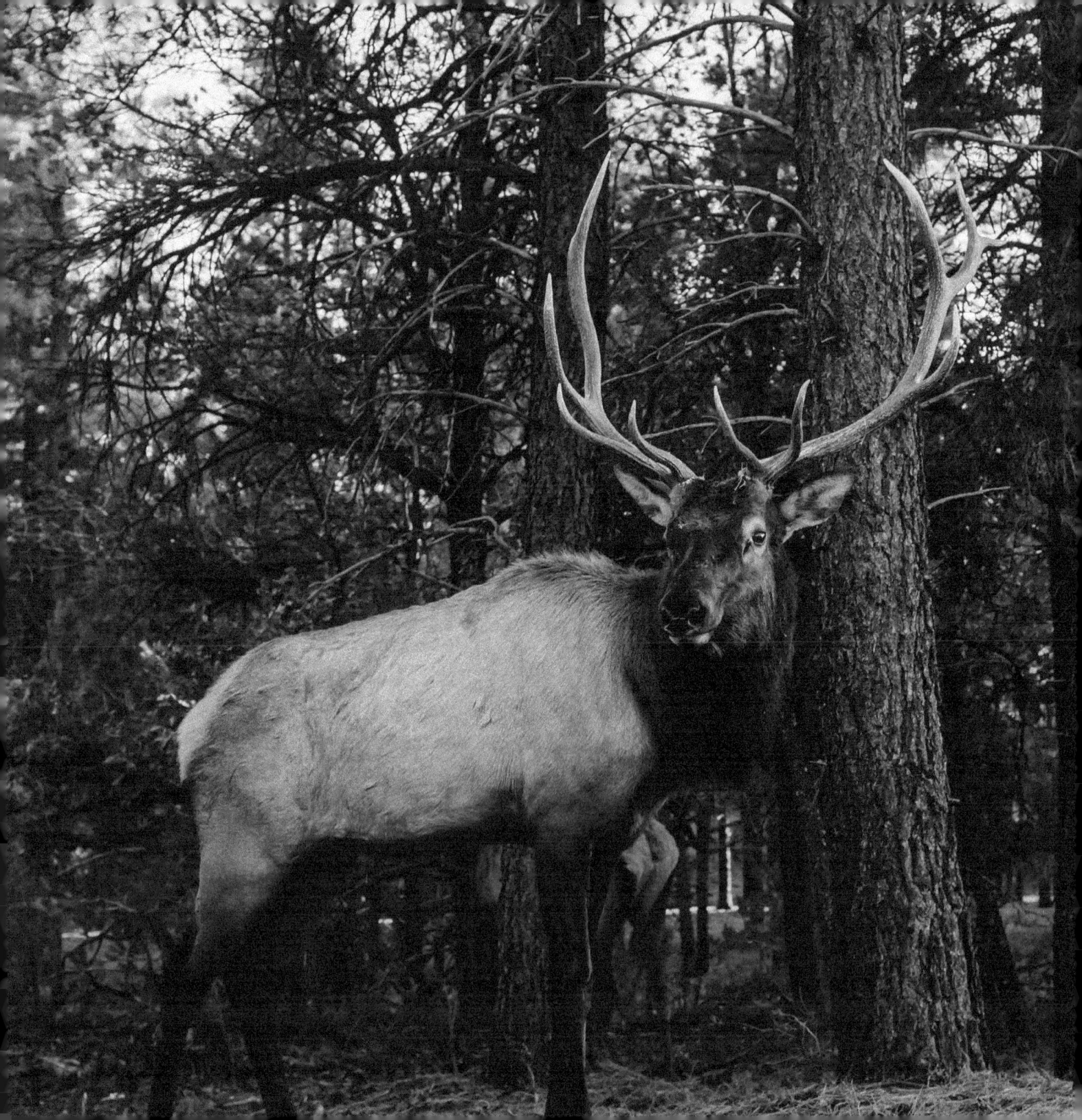

"Fighting to preserve our mind...is only possible with the greatest of alertness."
-
VENERABLE CHWASAN

Preserve your mind.

Take note: this is not referring to keeping intact cognition (crucial as that is). Rather, Venerable Chwasan describes how lust, greed, and comfort—amongst other desires—are continually trying to steal our minds away.

The quiet mind, the one we are in control of, the one we can notice, have kindness for, focus easily, and see Truth within… It's an attractive target.

If we let our guard down, we may just slip. We may just lose our agency over it.

In his book *The Principle of Training the Mind*, the former head dharma master states that the "wisest people are those who watch their health when they are healthy… cultivate their fields well when weeds are…scarce". The only path toward this preservation is to train the mind in awareness, to have the wisdom and courage to recognize and fend off the thieving desires. In practice, this might be intrusive thoughts of media images damaging our vision of ourselves. This might look like the pursuit of material goods clouding how we think or who we want to become. It's unending.

We train our minds to these ends via meditation. And as I'll state again and again, this can look a lot of different ways. It can take many shapes and be of various durations.

Like any training meant to strengthen, it requires consistency.

You show up and you show up and you show up again, expecting nothing day to day.

Cultivate your plentiful field. And heck, if yours is earthen scarcity, cultivate with more rigor and more self-directed kindness and love. Not unlike other skilled domains (whether sport, art, craft, or even human kinship), training harder here is all about frequency and effort as much as it is about the quality of our attention and intention.

Less pain, more gain.

"In the untrained mind there is ceaseless movement, filled with plans, ideas, and memories. Seeing this previously unconscious stream of inner dialogue is one of the first insights in meditation practice."

-

JOSEPH GOLDSTEIN, JACK KORNFIELD

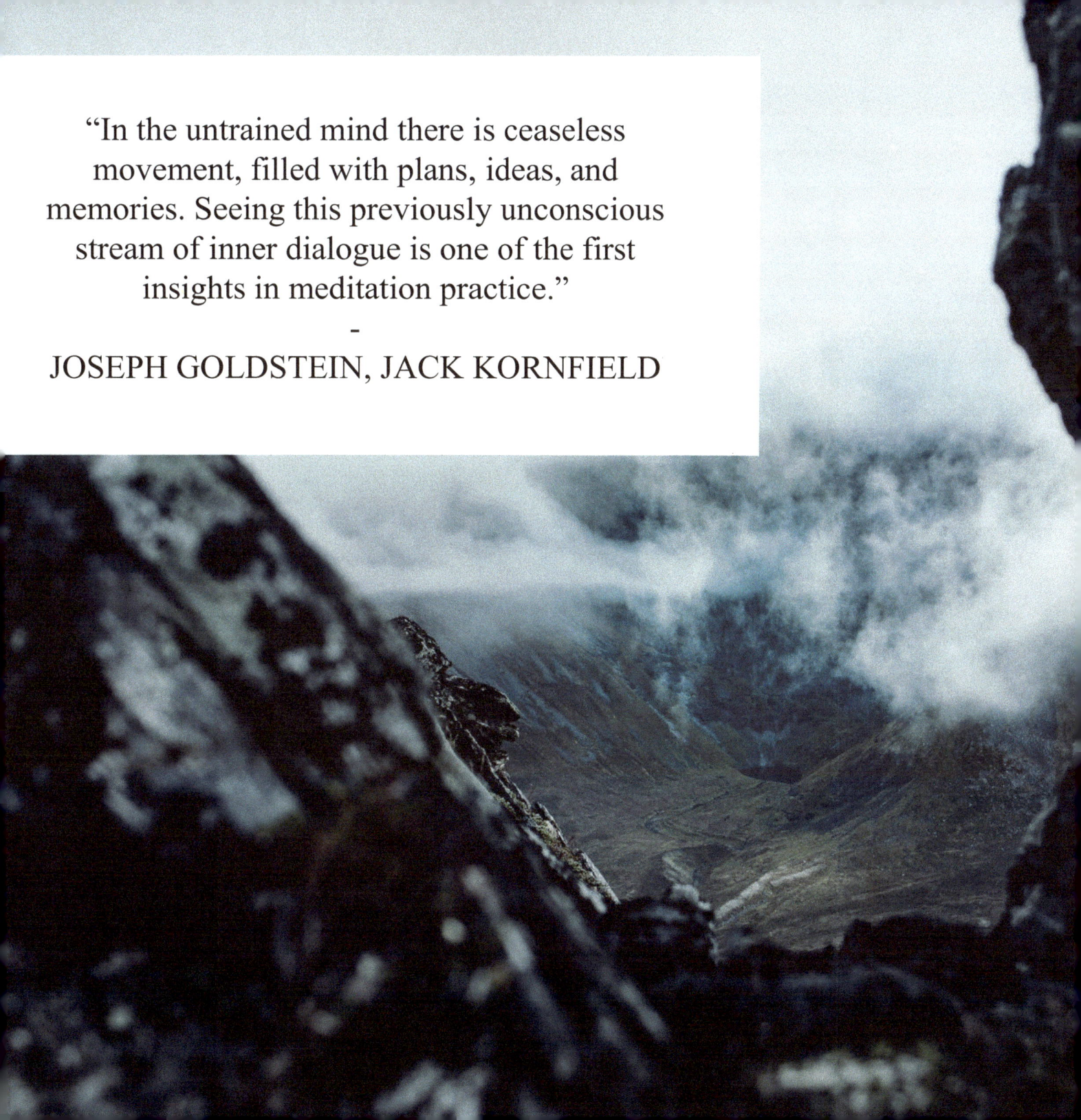

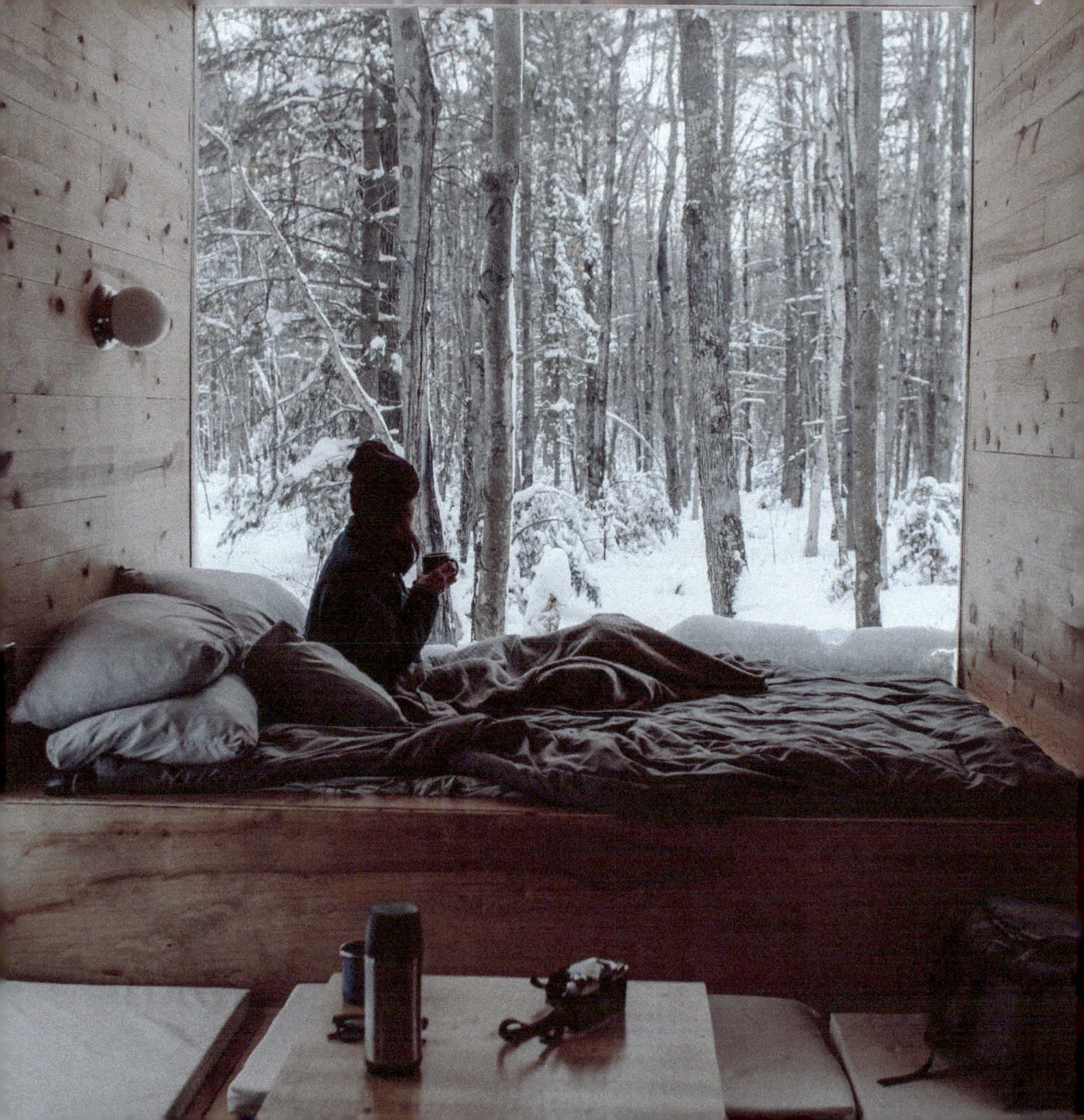

"We have never stayed home long enough
to experience the truth about ourselves."
-
ERICH SCHIFFMANN

Although "home" here describes something much less literal, can we not take both senses of the word to serious heart? What if we heeded the call to stay home, times two?

1. What if we took a moment to experience what exists inside of our houses that we have not noticed nor attended to in a long while? Inside the homes and out in the gardens we've built for ourselves and our families, upon which we've spent countless dollars and hours to achieve a Goldilocks-right feel.

- The abundance, the allowances, the physical space, noise, and silence... the sometimes stir-crazy children or frazzled adults, the dusty books, the recipes, the Netflix, the mail orders, the board games, the blessed, blessed boredom. Need we always, "get away"?

2. And what might happen if we took a moment to experience coming home to ourselves via slowing down, taking pause, being deliberate about reflection and meditation, in whatever form?

- What do we see, hear, feel, get a sense of, when we get quiet for longer than usual?

- What might we find if we allowed ourselves to go further, past the check-in marker we normally practice, if any?

- What if we got curious about our personal truth and our collective one?

Come home. Stay home. Relish.

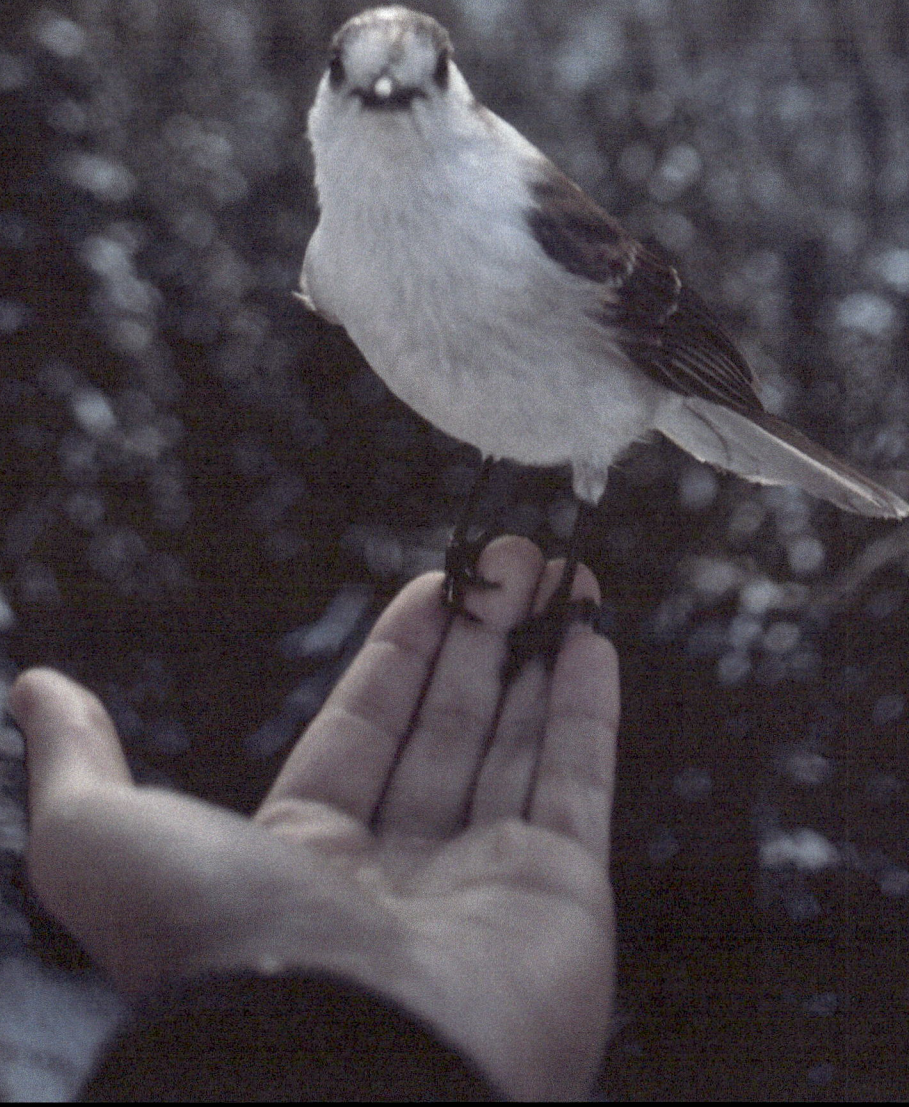

"The next message you need is always right where you are."
-
RAM DASS

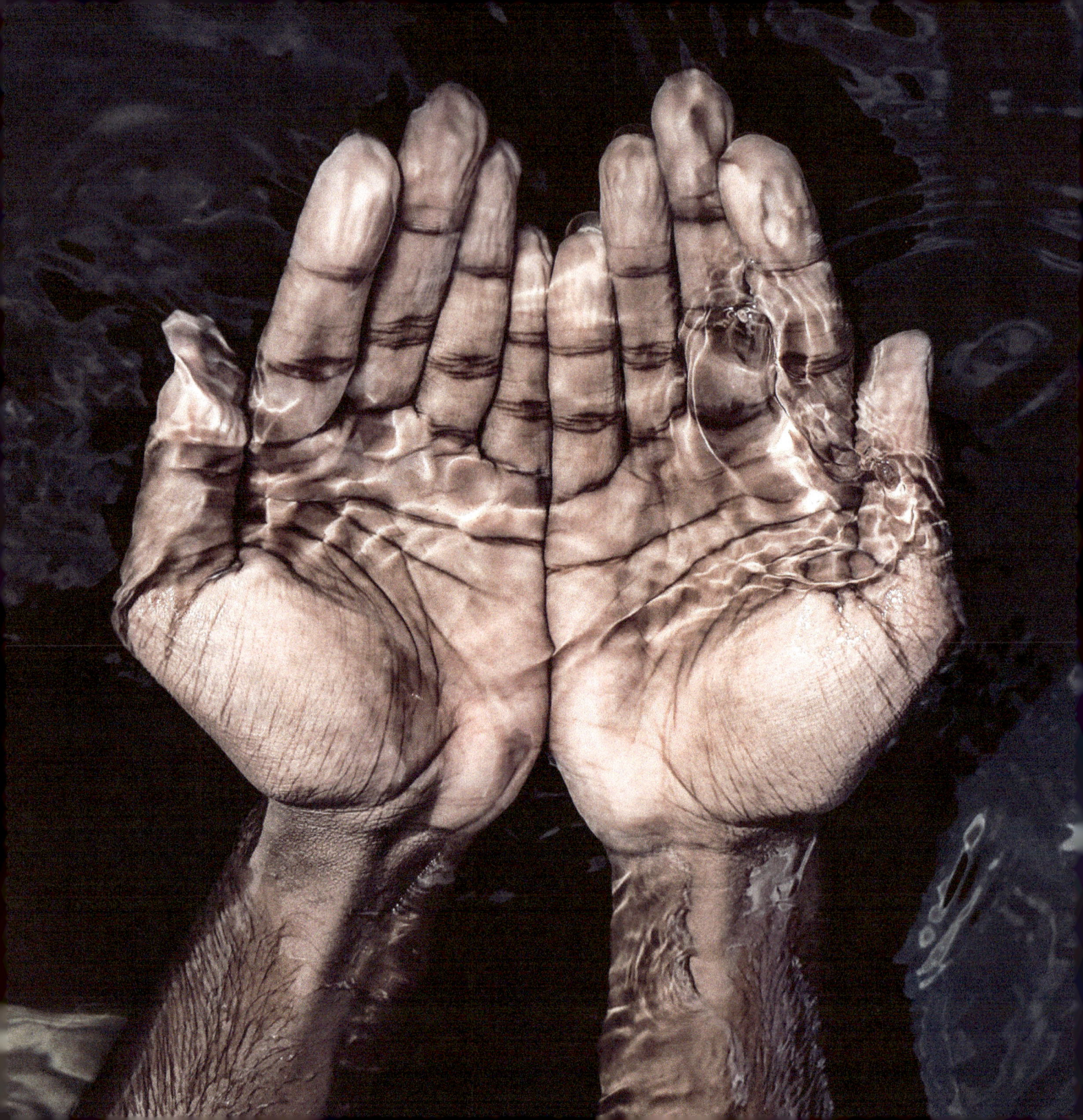

"Everything happens for you,
not to you."
-
BYRON KATIE

This quotation changed my life.

I'm not joking.

Take a minute. Use this in application to any number of challenges you are personally facing. See if it doesn't change the way you view everything. One short phrase equaling total perspective shift, in an instant. One short but *huge*, weighty word: that "for".

If truly understood as something given to us, something meant to serve us, might we be able to gather some insight from an issue, rather than allow it to do us harm?

With just this simple but profound wording, "this is happening *for* me," we are instantly allowed to drop our sense of victimhood—to just take that coat right off—and are reborn. We realize that life is challenge and overcoming; it's wild with peaks and valleys. And it's ALL *for* us.

Can we appreciate the enormous offering?

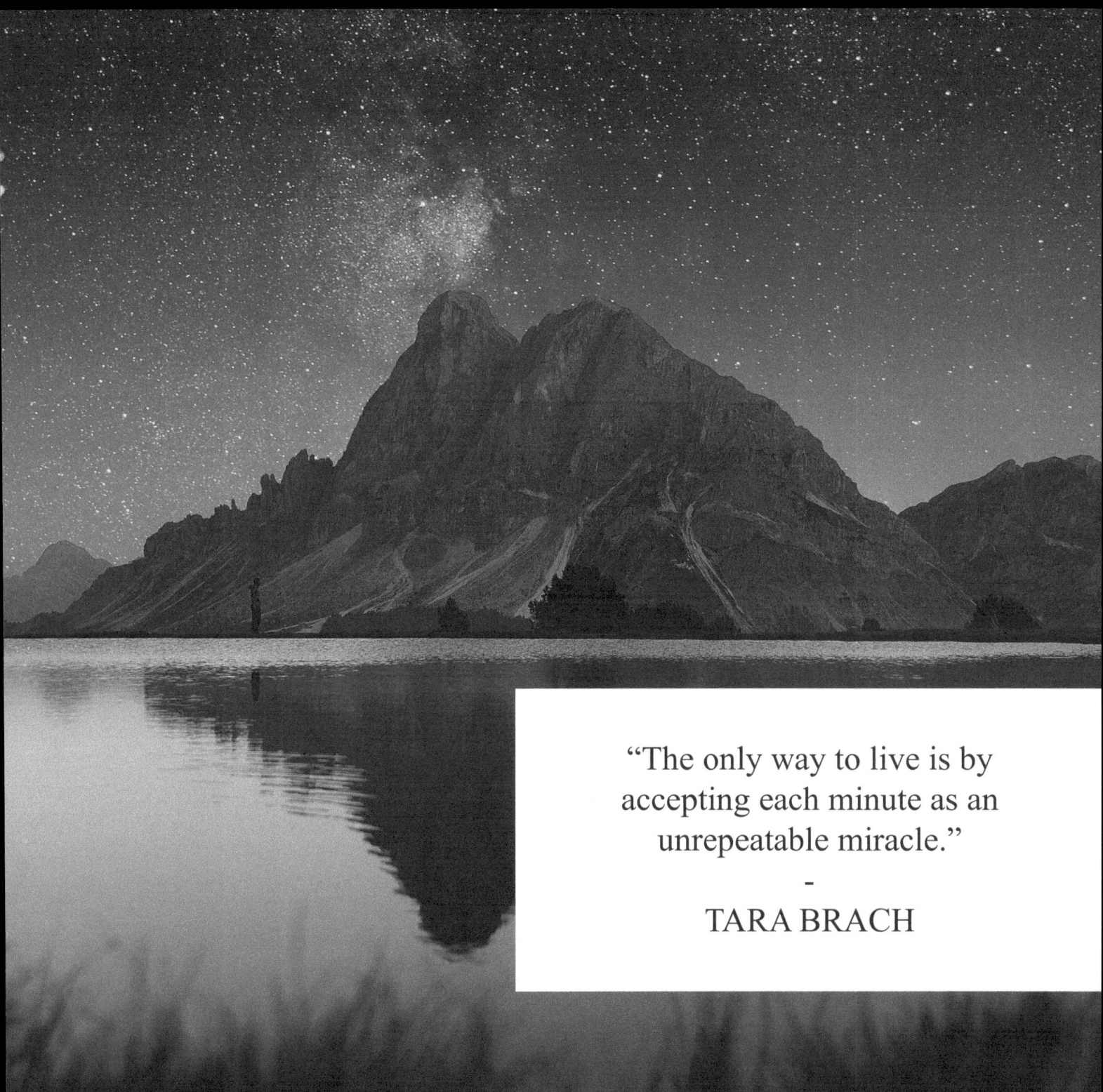

"The only way to live is by accepting each minute as an unrepeatable miracle."

-

TARA BRACH

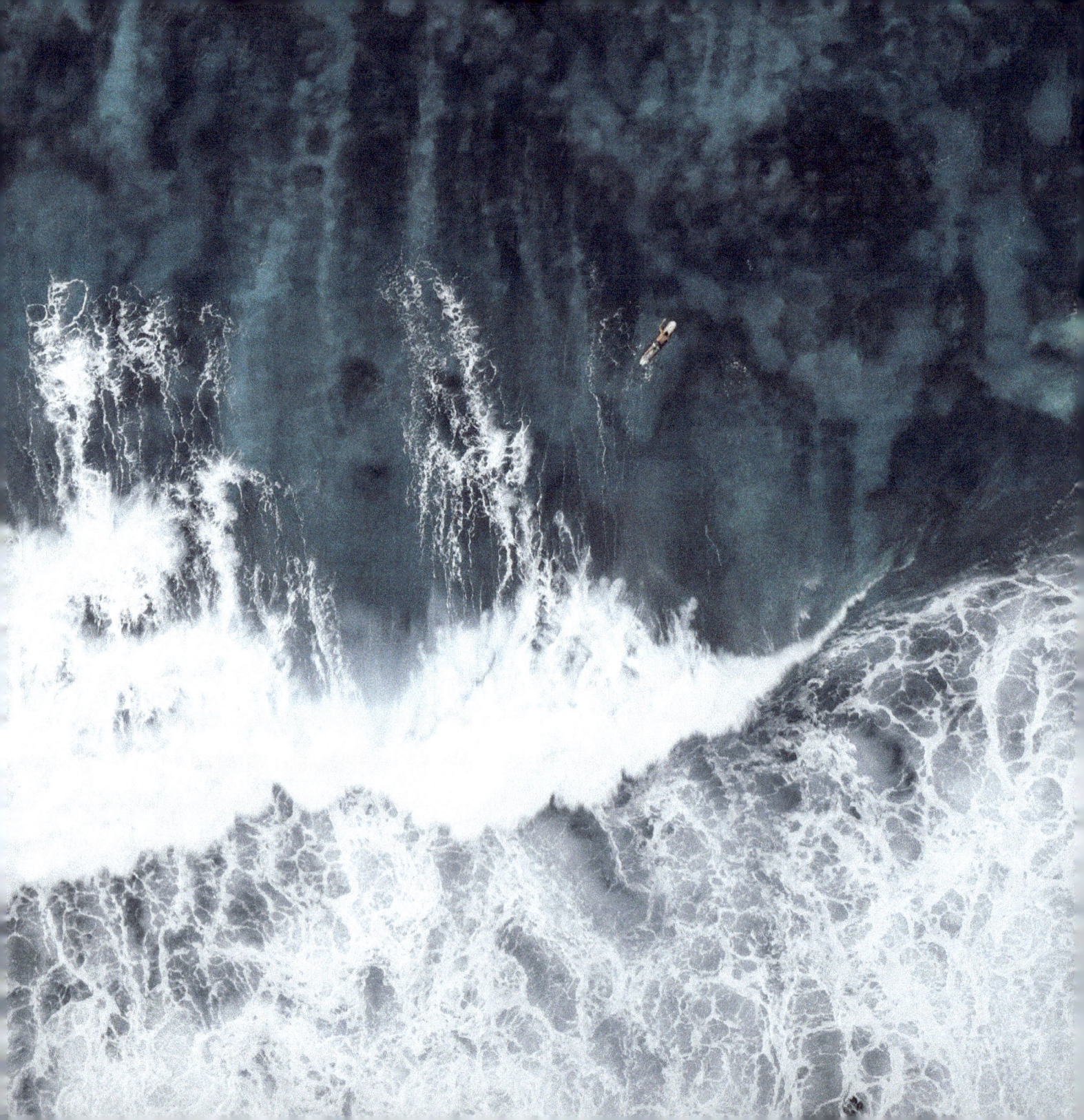

"Our actions almost always correspond to dispositions of mind. When I am impatient, traffic moves too slowly; when I am angry, others are irritating; when consumed and preoccupied with myself, other people only get in the way... This means that we don't need to wait around for the culture to change—the imbalances right in front of our eyes are laid out like freshly stretched canvases."

-

MICHAEL STONE

On the days when everything feels topsy turvy, I come back to this. When there is an overwhelming sense of anxiety and fear in the world, it's a good visual to recall. While turning outward in kindness is in desperate need, we must understand that if we skip the inward part, we will lose all ability to paint that canvas artfully. In those moments, we need our mind-body practices strengthened more than ever.

It is time to become aware of our disposition and to get in touch with how our inner state either clouds or clears our judgment. It is time to cultivate (or to strengthen commitment to cultivating) our minds and spirits via the uncomplicated tools of yoga, meditation, and mindfulness.

The first thing is to stop making excuses.

We must ask ourselves if we want our view of the world around us to change for the better.

Would we like our experience to lighten?

What Stone is telling us here is that it starts with us, and it starts within. Just as we were told as children, we are all artists.

"Your life doesn't get any better than your mind is: You might have wonderful friends, perfect health, a great career, and everything else you want, and you can still be miserable. The converse is also true: There are people who basically have nothing—who live in circumstances that you and I would do more or less anything to avoid—who are happier than we tend to be because of the character of their minds. Unfortunately, one glimpse of this truth is never enough. We have to be continually reminded of it."

-

SAM HARRIS

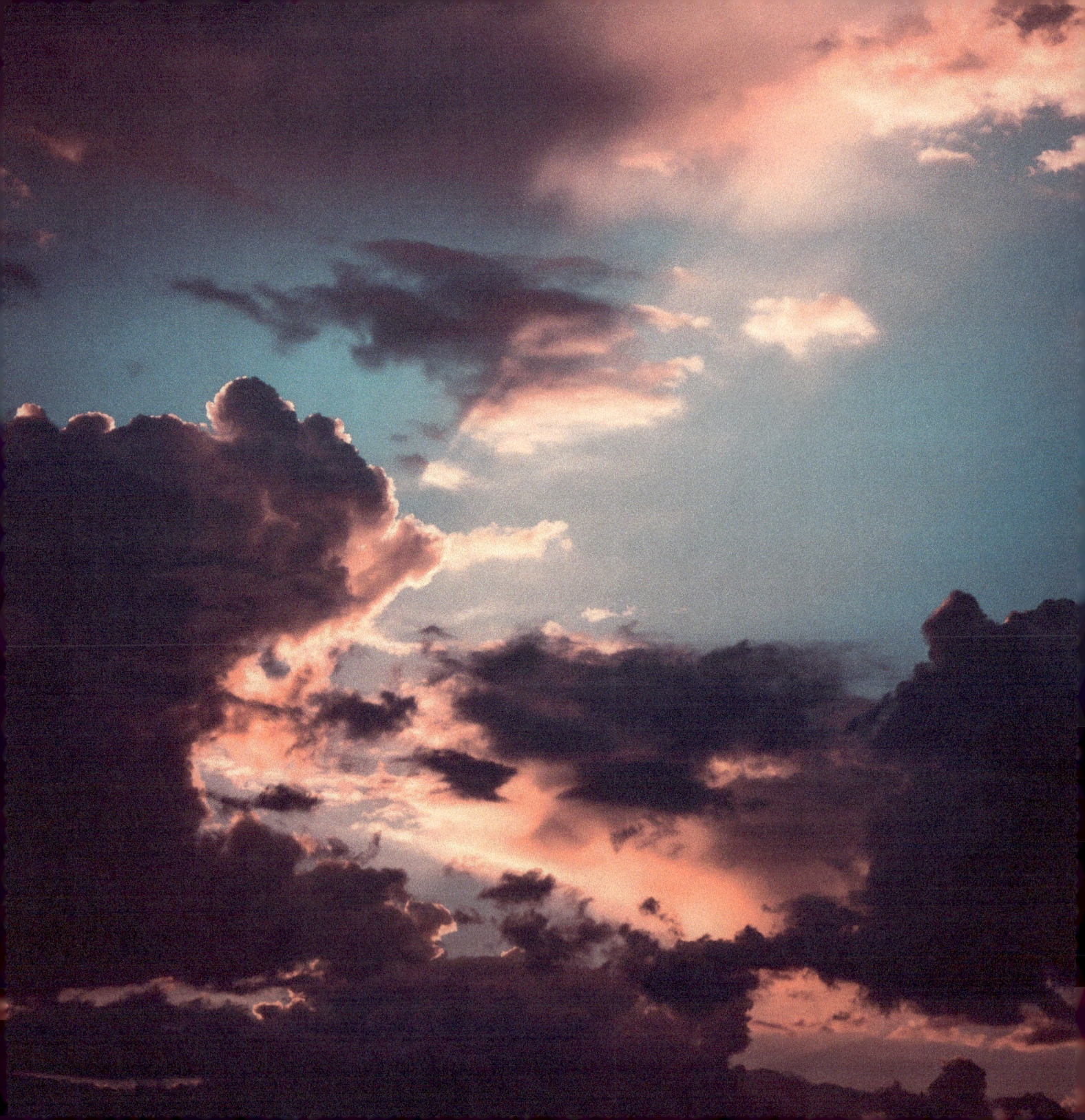

"You are the sky—everything else,
it's just the weather."
-
PEMA CHODRON

You are the sky.

Ugh. So strikingly beautiful.

I cannot imagine a better, more fitting metaphor for the self and observation of the self than this.

How are we ever to see or approximate knowing our true nature if all we ever experience are our fluctuant moods? You are not your ups and downs. You are not your shining moments as a human just as much as you are not your rock-bottoms.

When you look outside, try erasing the weather. To be able to see who/what we really are, we have to acquire this skill. And while this might seem an impossible riddle or one of those 3D art pieces that most of us will never visualize (even if we squint until our faces hurt), it's about as simple as this: Picture the sky. Remove any other veils from view.

No one ever confused the immensity, wonder, beauty, complexity, or simplicity of the sky with cloud or fog or sun or rain.

The first step to knowing yourself is this.

If you are lacking confidence or wading in self-judgment or beating yourself up over something you said or did or didn't say or didn't do, I'm here to remind you: you are the sky.

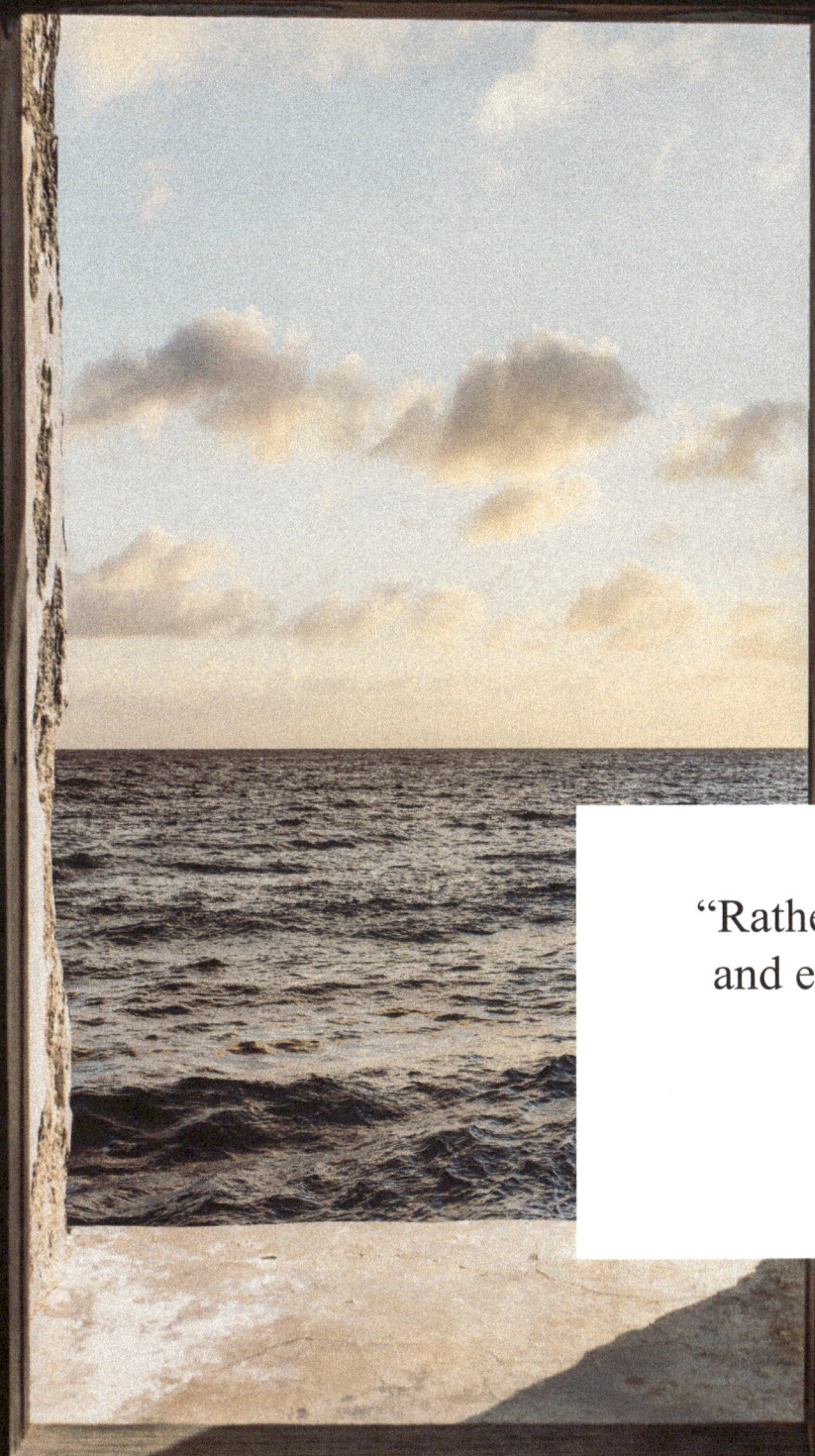

"Rather than being your thoughts and emotions, be the awareness behind them."

-

ECKHART TOLLE

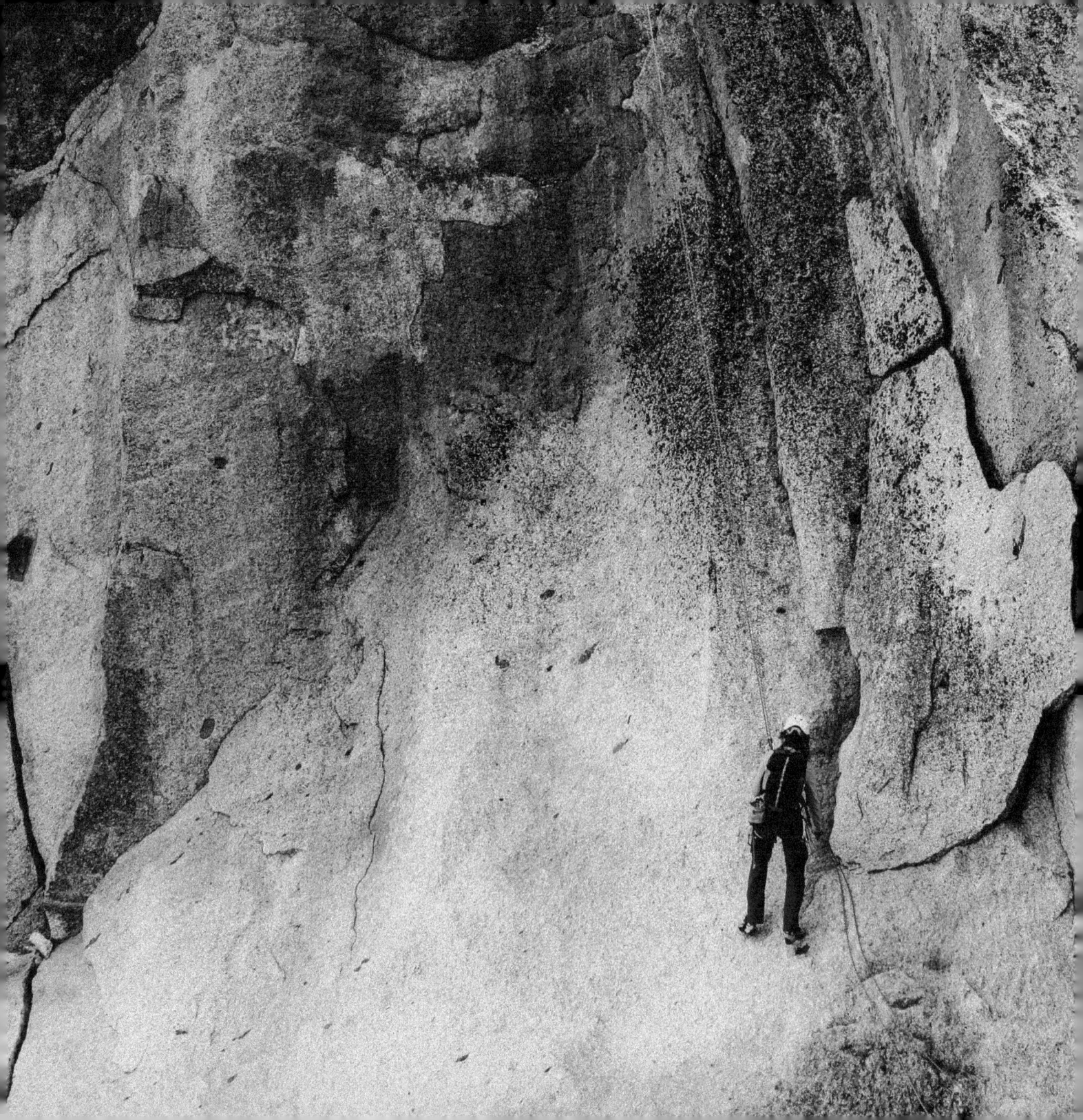

"I believe that attention is the singular most important asset for anybody trying to achieve anything."

-

GARY VAYNERCHUK
(GARY VEE)

Attention.

Pretty captivating.

Where is your attention focused these days?

If you are trying to gain more clients, grow a following, pivot your business, upon what or where are you placing your attention resources? Are your eyes on the proverbial prize?

Whether your aim is self-improvement, reversing physical/emotional dis-ease or health optimization, is your attention laser focused on that very aim? Or are you caught up? Are you researching the thing, are you stuck in peripherals, in daily minutiae that don't move your needle forward in any particular way? In yoga there is a saying: Look where you want to go. If you're in a balancing posture and your eyes are focused on the ground, rest assured you'll end up there.

If your attention is placed upon what you're trying to avoid, it is as simple as shifting your gaze toward what you actually want.

You'll see that it starts with this gaze, the one attentive to and intent upon your primary goal. And from there, everything else shifts in that direction, naturally. Your entire frame. Your being.

Today, right now. Be intentional about your attention.

"It is the power to focus the consciousness on a given spot, and hold it there. Attention is the first and indispensable step in all knowledge. "

-

PATAÑJALI

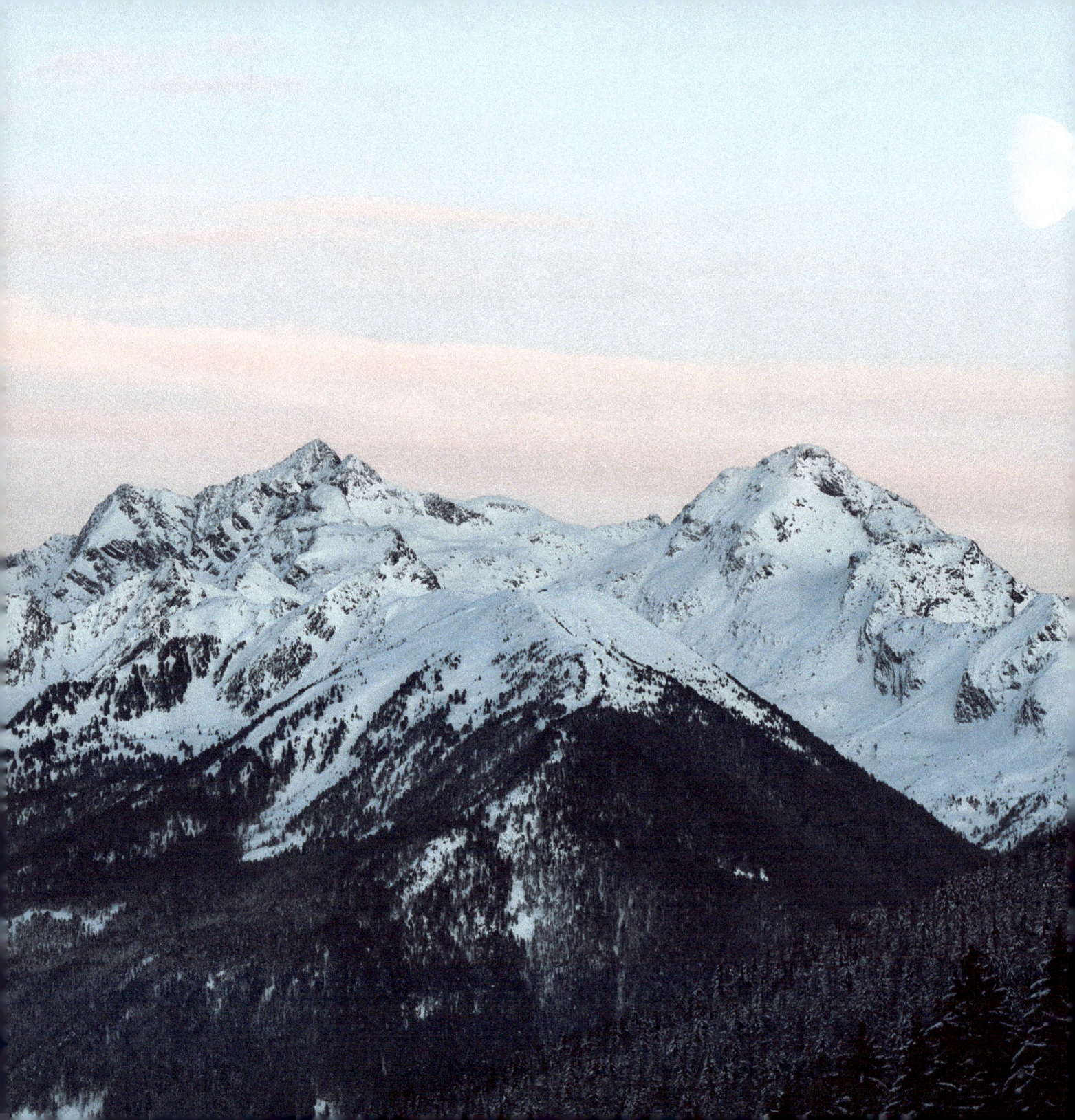

"The real meditation is
how you live your life."
-
JON KABAT-ZINN

You may be wondering why anyone would find capital M "Meaning" in a practice that involves sitting for minutes or hours each day, focused on…well not much of anything.

What JKZ says here is your answer. When we practice—be this yoga, mindfulness, meditation, attention, whatever—our aim and answered call is always a life enriched by the same elements that make you go "aaaahh" after a blissful little practice.

When we are *consistent* with our chosen practice, small bits every day, and we are genuine within it (the difference between holding your breath in a pose and breathing it), its benefits inevitably seep through into everyday life. This is what is meant by yoga "off the mat," or life being a "walking meditation."

At some point, when our bodies and brains are patterned in the same way, again and again through gentle, conscious effort, the hours and minutes between practice blur, fade, and eventually, disappear. We can no longer separate waking life from these moments of practice. It's bliss.

But also… That life really is the true test. It's easy to breathe deeply and get conscious, be gentle and at our most considerate when in silence and unbothered and calm. Where we're challenged and tested is in the Monday mornings at work and the Thursday night bedtime routines.

Where we can really see if we're getting the point at all, is in the sticky, normal, frustrating, ugly, routine moments of daily life. When we ask ourselves, have we learned enough to truly live it?

Read this quote again.

This is why we practice.

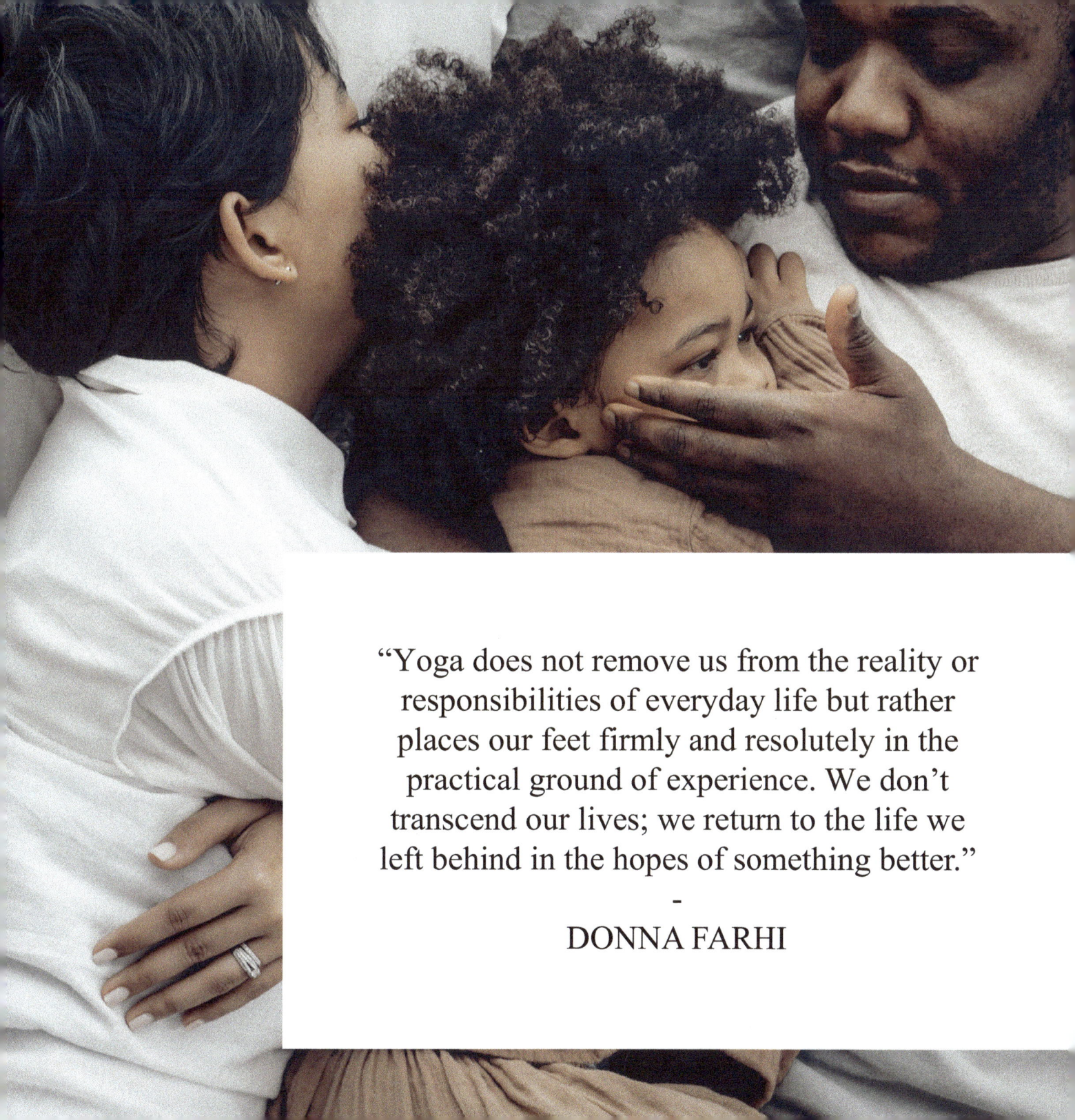

"Yoga does not remove us from the reality or responsibilities of everyday life but rather places our feet firmly and resolutely in the practical ground of experience. We don't transcend our lives; we return to the life we left behind in the hopes of something better."

-

DONNA FARHI

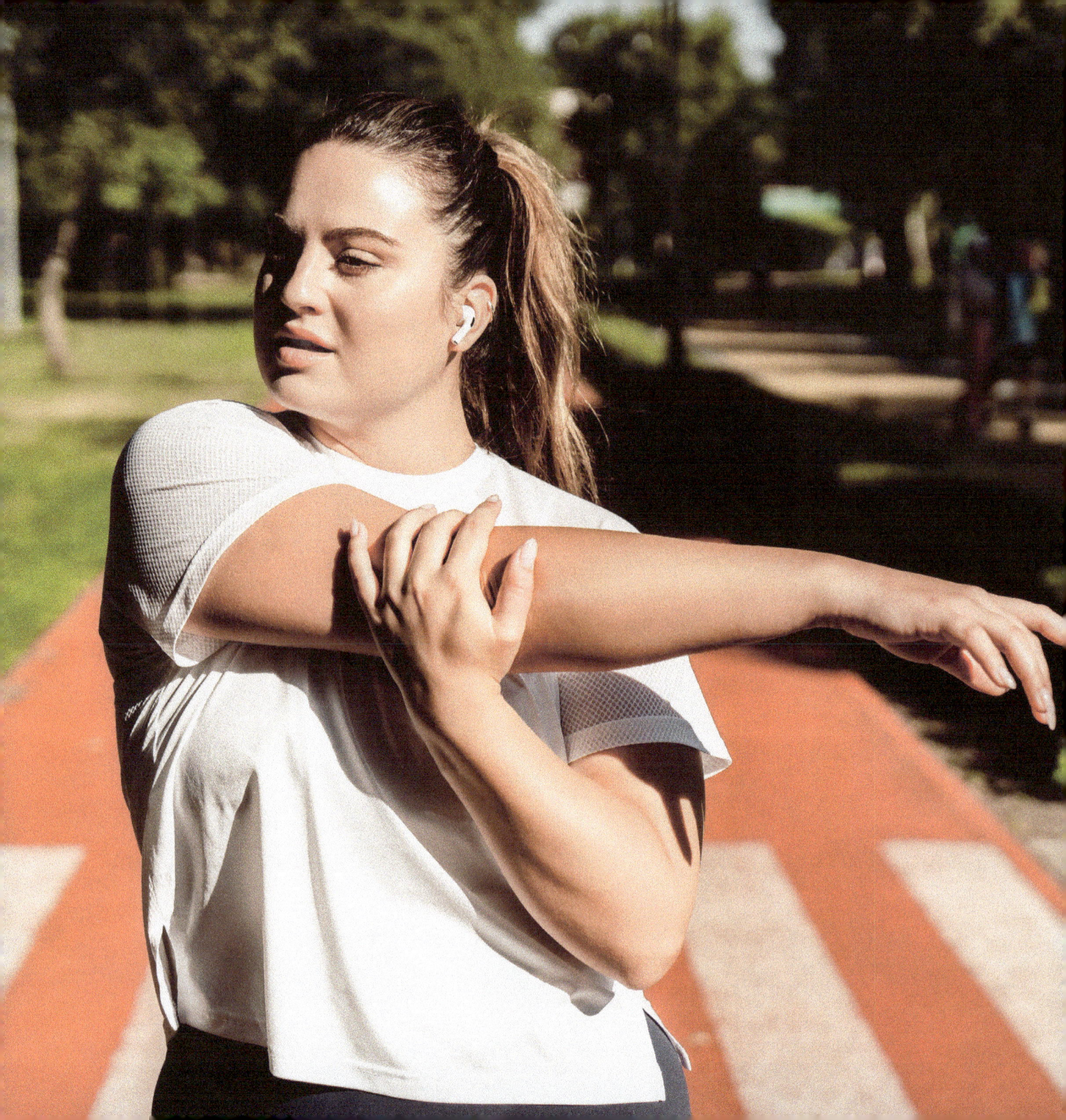

"Move a muscle,
change a feeling."
-
UNKNOWN

How about, *move a few?*

Any which way you like.

I used to teach English to second language learners. My number one piece of advice, when they approached me after class asking how to accelerate their learning, was to consume the language in the way they most enjoyed. Love fiction? Pick up a few books and devour them. Hip hop is your thing? Have English-speaking artists playing constantly in your earbuds and read a few lyrics when you can. If you (even halfway) enjoy the process, your outcomes will far outpace and outweigh those hating every second of their worksheets.

Certainly, I'm not dropping any novel wisdom by telling you that moving your body will hugely benefit your mind, mood, and so many other aspects of your well-being.

This is meant as a reminder that when you choose to engage in some sort of physical activity (especially one you enjoy) you will immediately change how you feel for the better. Instant and lasting results. Available to you anywhere, anytime. For free. Which at the same time, does a zillion things for your physiological health.

I want you to check in with your many excuses: I don't have time, I'm watching my kids, I'm not strong or skilled or whatever you're telling yourself. Find those excuses

and then ask yourself, "So I don't have time/energy/strength...to feel better?".

Don't you?

Choose to.

Move. Your. Body.

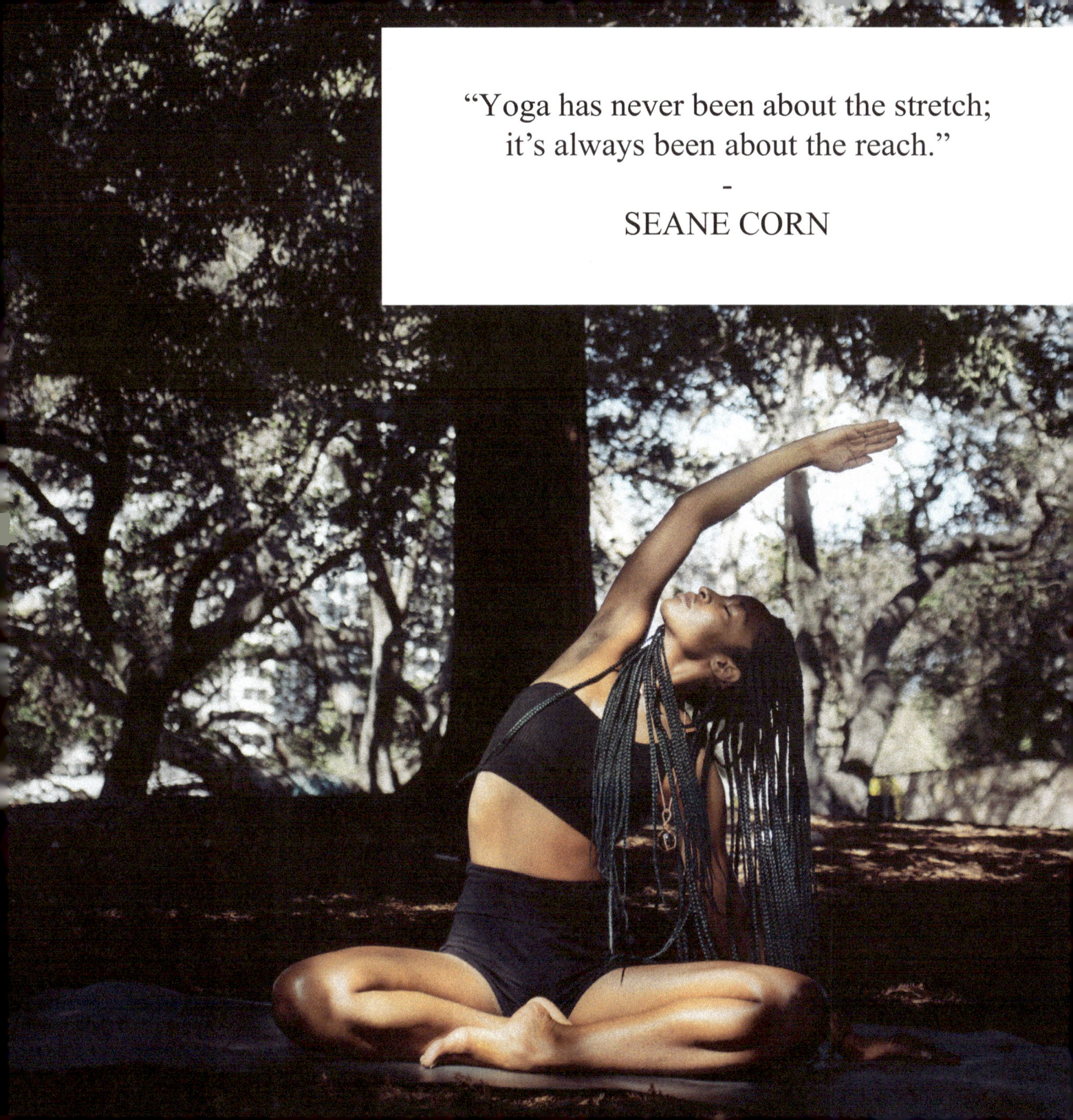

"Yoga has never been about the stretch;
it's always been about the reach."
-
SEANE CORN

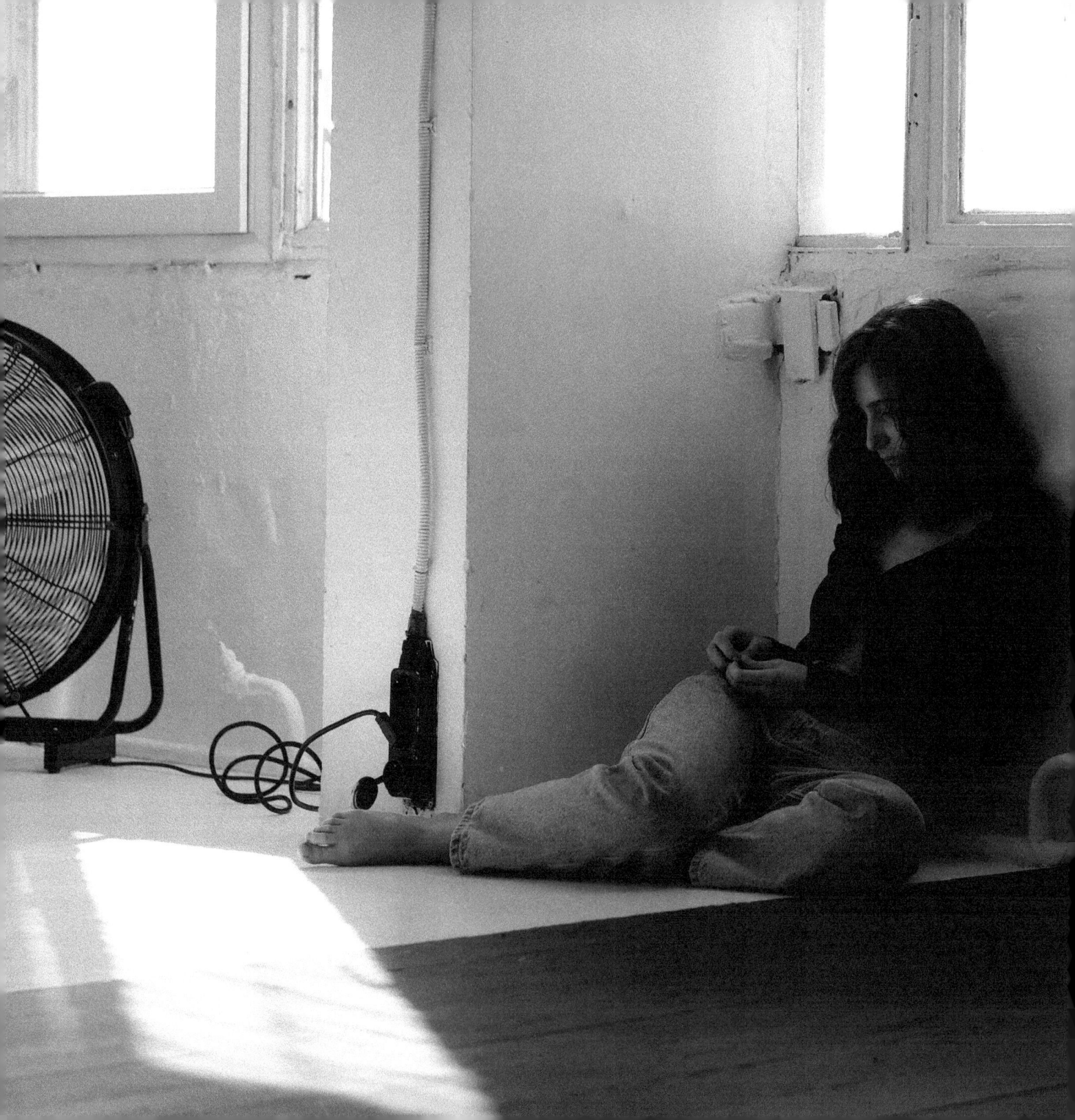

"Sometimes you need to sit lonely
on a floor in a quiet room in order to
hear your own voice and
not let it drown in the noise of others."

-

CHARLOTTE ERIKSSON

Ever felt this way?

It's funny, I used to think I was an extrovert. Needing the outlet of friends, family, gatherings, or one-on-ones...the "social." And while there's no question we are a social species (and I'm not excluded from this), as I grow, I am finding I need ever increasing amounts of quiet.

That quiet isn't always meditation or yoga. It's true that sometimes quiet really is about silencing or slowing down thoughts and inner dialogue. But sometimes, it's about lowering the volume on all things outer noise. That is, allowing your own beautiful, creative, mile-a-minute brain to do its thing while you: drive/sit/walk/run/journal/listen to music/dance/look out the window.

Leaving the judgments, ideas, advice, and suggestions of others (however well meaning) at the doorstep and closing the door to a glorious, just-you, sort of epic quiet.

I have found this to be immensely nourishing. Especially, when in a time of transition and growth.

Can you hear yourself think?

Close the door. Enter that quiet space.

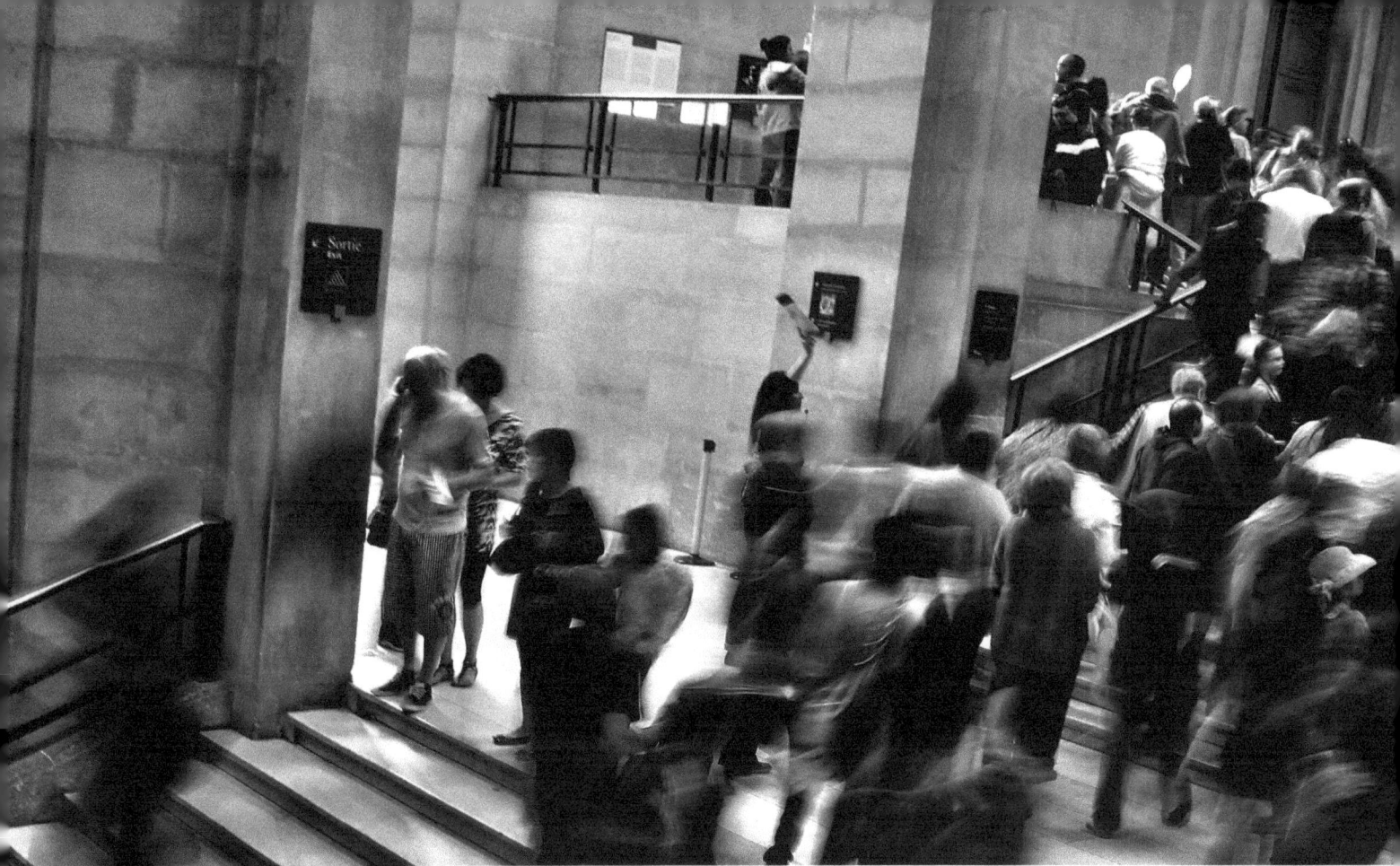

"If we feed ourselves noise on a regular basis,
until we don't even recognize it as noise,
how can we expect to quiet the mind?"
-

MAX STROM

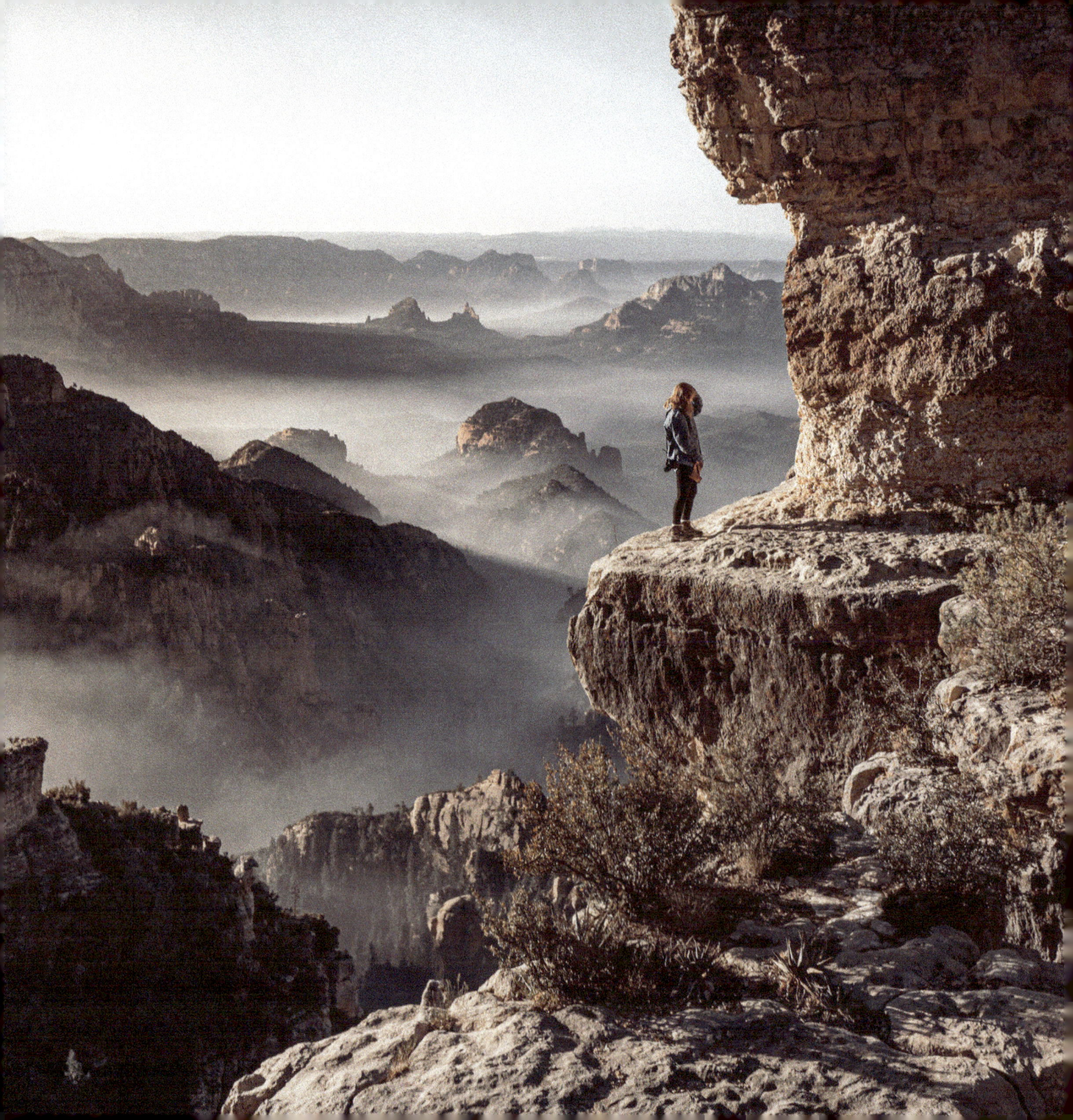

"Endure both
[the good and the bad],
whichever arises."

-

GESHE KELSANG GYATSO

"Endure both, whichever arises." In his book, *Universal Compassion*, Geshe Kelsang Gyatso breaks this little piece of Buddhist scripture down in a digestible way.

Essentially this: Take both positive and negative life circumstances and accept them. Accept them in a way that prevents either from getting in the way of your spiritual practice. One which, instead, helps to develop that practice further.

Of course, it's easy to imagine how a demanding or painful moment could be the proverbial quicksand in our path—easy to fall off course, off practice, off faith. But the good times? Our worldly wins and highs?

Imagine winning the lottery. How likely are you, a few months later, to keep journaling your gratitudes? To treat everyone the exact same way you used to? To appreciate the small things that used to mean a lot? Possible, but without proper grounding, not likely.

You don't have to win a ridiculous amount of money for a happy circumstance to take you off course. On the days following a promotion, an accomplishment, or some great news, do you rush to meditate? Or to read or pray or do the work that you know nurtures your soul?

Endure both, whichever arises.

That is to say, embrace both. Use them well. Don't get lost.

"Accept—then act. Whatever the present moment contains, accept it as if you had chosen it. Always work with it, not against it…This will miraculously transform your whole life."

-

ECKHART TOLLE

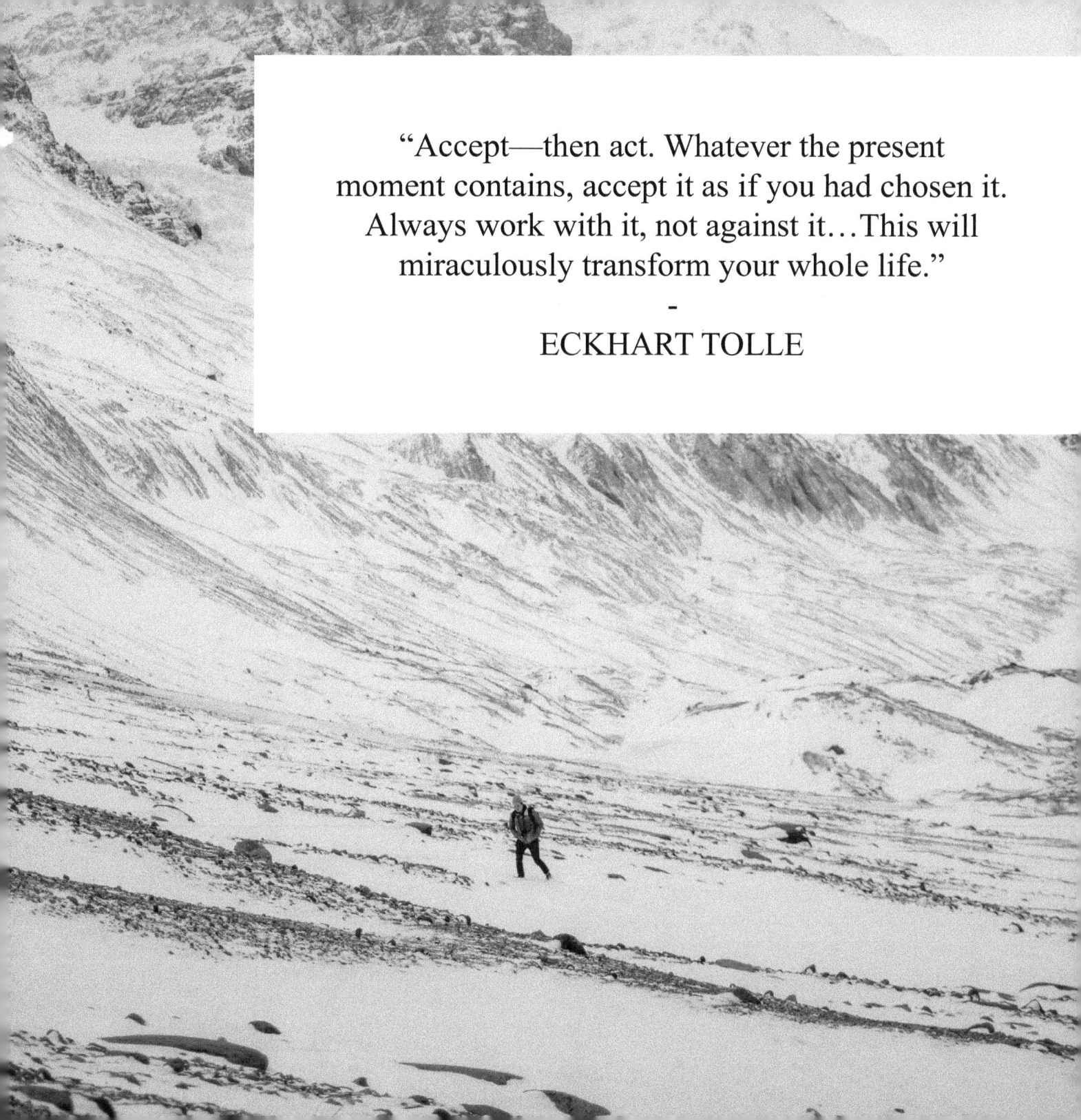

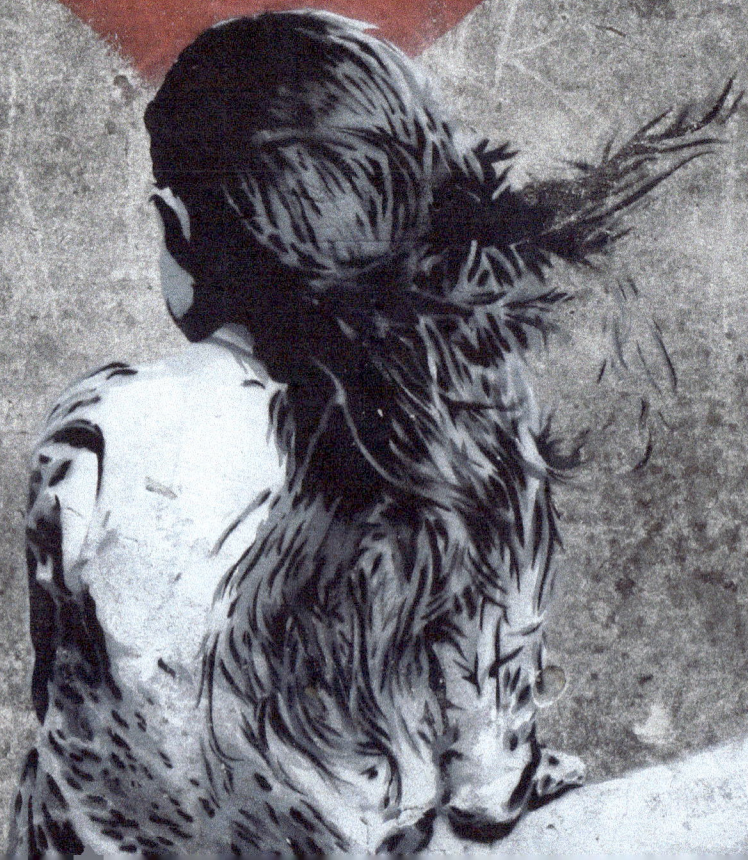

"An intellectual mind that is unconnected to the heart is an uncultivated mind."

-

BKS IYENGAR

Two giants. The heart and the mind... For some reason, at least in North American society, we place so much more value on that brain/mind thing. Trust me, I value it highly, too. Expanding and strengthening one's intellect is synonymous with evolution. What distinguishes us from the Cro-Magnon and everything before and in between.

Though we used to think a larger brain meant smarter, scientists now know that while that was an earlier evolutionary trend, in the past few tens of thousands of years, our brains have actually been getting smaller and more efficient rather than less intelligent. And while we generally continue to praise brains over emotional or intuitive brawn, have we unwittingly weakened and devalued that unthinking part of us that feels?

Now before you jump all over me with lectures re: the nervous system and the emotional warehouses of the brain—I get it. It's absolutely true that without our brain we wouldn't feel or be able to process sensation or emotion of any sort.

What I'm trying to describe is the *heart* of which Iyengar here speaks. We understand that he's not referring to that thing with four chambers which pumps our blood and keeps us ticking. We also understand that he's not quite referring to the amygdala.

So, what is this elusive heart we are urged to grasp, in order to cultivate our minds?

In fact, the heart of this quotation may well be the mind we refer to when we talk about meditation, about mindfulness, about our own spiritual awareness, growth, and development. We must be able to properly distinguish the words "brain," "intellect," and "mind" as very distinct things, though that last one isn't so easy to pin down.

Decide for yourself where compassion, empathy, love, and kindness reside.

I want to raise a child with strong intellect but even stronger ♥.

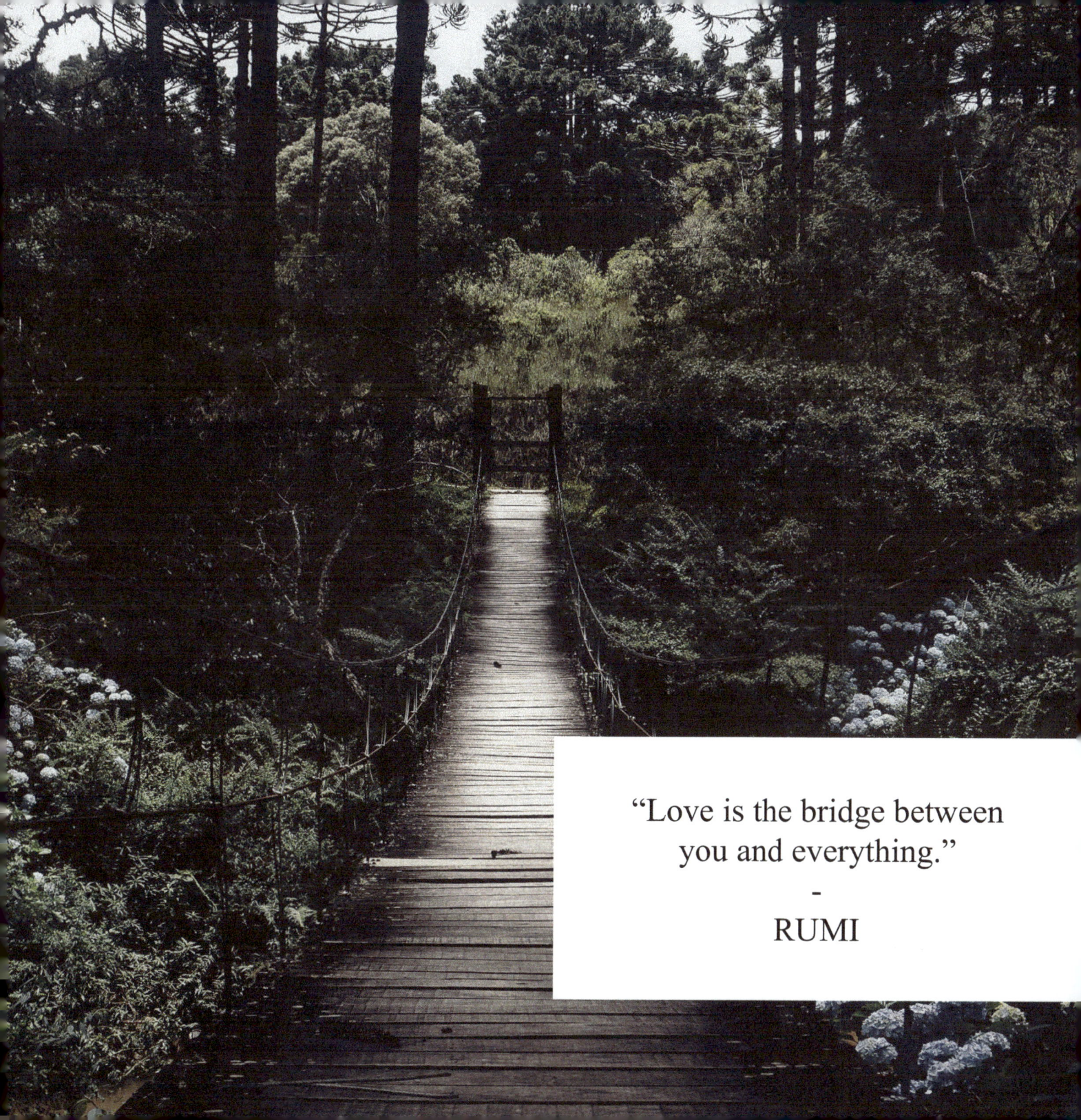

"Love is the bridge between
you and everything."
-

RUMI

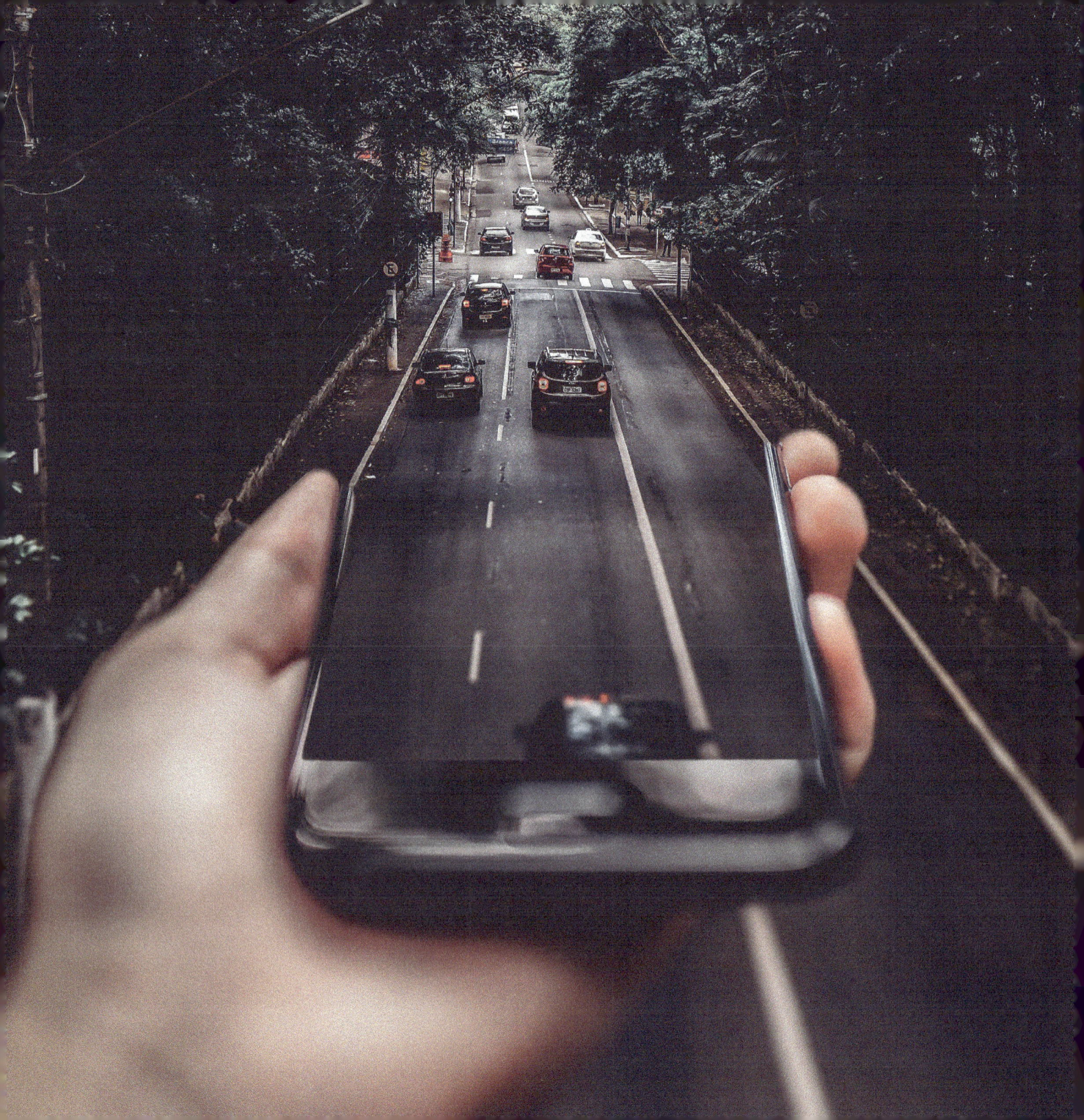

"You should sit in meditation for twenty minutes a day—unless you're too busy; then you should sit for an hour."

-

UNKNOWN

Does this make you smile? Or make you raving mad? The notion that we who are too busy should have to devote *more* of our time. What nerve, Zen Masterunknown!

So, is this tongue in cheek? Or is this an actual (however unnerving) prescription for time on our seats?

Well, the best answer is, both.

Yes, it's playful. Yes, it pokes at how we choose to prioritize our time in this age of fast-paced-everything. Rightly or wrongly, if we're honest, on a busy day, are we making time for slowing down? Are we placing "attention practice" or "mindful awareness" near the top of that to-do list?

Of course, this aphorism isn't really asking us to sit for a whopping sixty minutes daily...right?
I wish I were joking, but, sort of.

In yoga circles, it is said that the pose that you hate, the one you avoid at all costs, is the one you need the most. This is *always* the case. We avoid that which is too strenuous, too uncomfortable, the one that shoots down our ego too much. And so, with life, and meditation.

Let's call out busyness for what it is (and trust me I'm speaking to my own reflection in the mirror here): It is a, rather full, series of tasks we have prioritized over others, which (from Merriam-Webster) "chiefly stresses activity as opposed to idleness or leisure."

Every soul on Earth has the same twenty-four hours and the same fifty-two weeks. Everyone is making their way, attending to their work, their families, their responsibilities. Why do some seem to always have the time, and others never? So, the mindset really does dictate the prescription. You feel the amount of activity you must accomplish in a day just doesn't allow for pause? That's your pose, friend. That's the one you have to sit and breathe in for longer than the rest. That's the one you have to stop avoiding.

We really don't and can't know what we're missing while we're missing it. Those that have never exercised will never understand how great it feels to push their bodies to the limits of their ability. Nor the powerful effect this can have on their lives. In the same way, those who have "no time" to meditate will never know just what they're missing.

Until they book that hour off.

"The pose begins when you want to get out of it."
-
BARON BAPTISTE,
quoting BKS IYENGAR

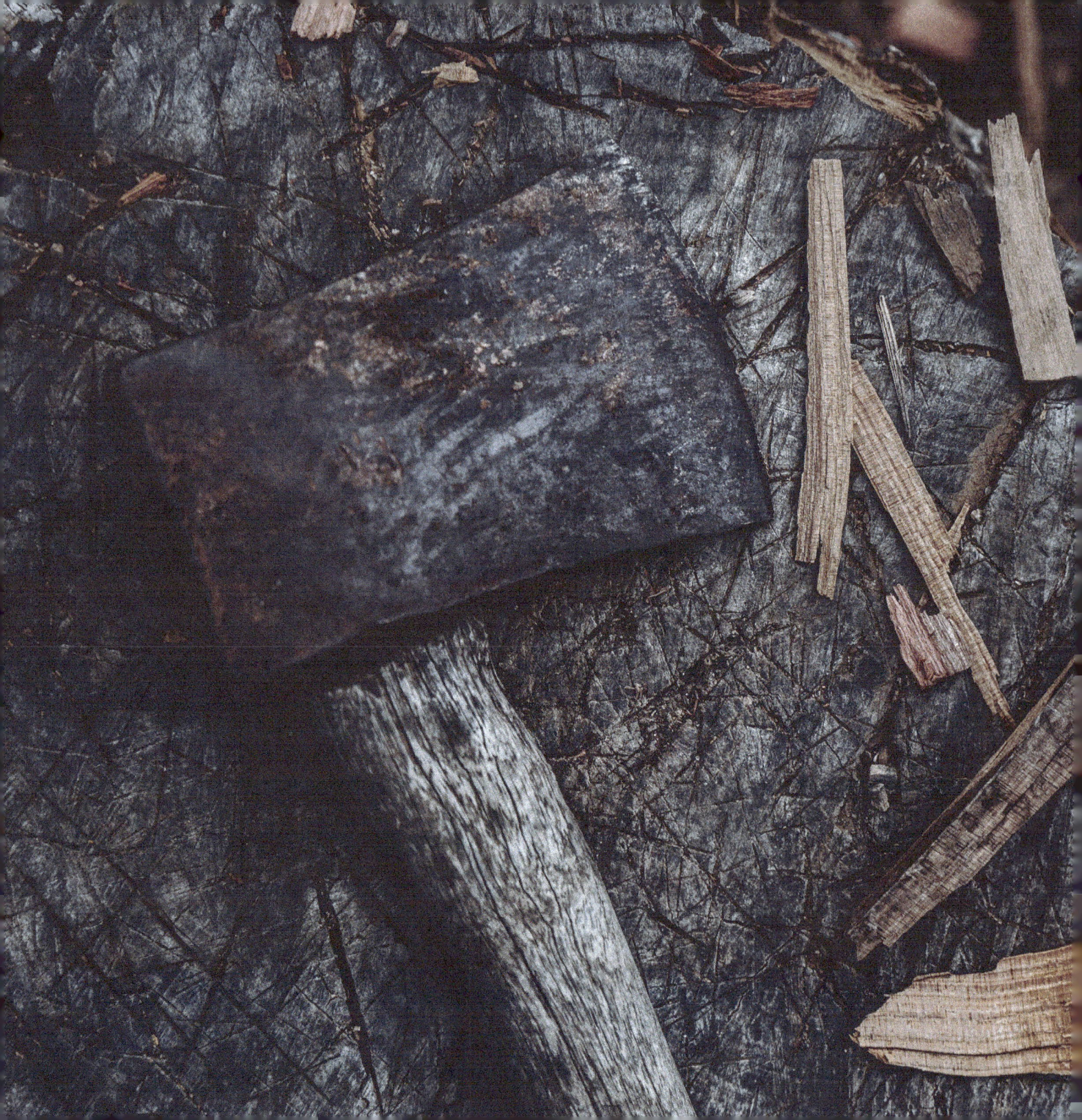

"Fill your bowl to the brim and it will spill. Keep sharpening your knife and it will blunt. Chase after money and security and your heart will never unclench. Care about people's approval and you will be their prisoner. Do your work, then step back. The only path to serenity."

-

LAO TZU
[translation by Steve Mitchell]

There's not much one can add to an excerpt from a work of genius. Lao Tzu's, *Book of the Way*, really does speak for itself.

What I can offer is something of mine, a story.

When I was staying in an ashram in the Kootenays some years ago, I learned one aspect of this last point about stepping back.

We were tasked with daily karma yoga duties. About eight hours a day of whatever work was assigned to us, broken up in two, four-hour chunks, separated by a lovely lunch. Karma yoga is about selfless action—essentially a type of volunteerism which is meant to benefit others whilst purifying one's soul on the path toward liberation. This work could take the form of anything from weeding flowerbeds, to folding linens, to cleaning urinals. One day, my morning shift had me washing heads of lettuce. Quite a few. We had a sort of assembly line set up, and I was near the end.

When the lunch bell rang, everyone around me immediately stopped what they were doing and made way for the dining area. I looked at the work remaining and kept at the job for a bit, thinking I'd make some headway on that lettuce.

Someone walking by noticed and called me out. "It's time for lunch." I responded with an explanation: There

seemed to be a lot of work, I would just do a bit more to complete my task. Don't we all love that feeling when we get to check that item off as "done?" How quickly I was shut down.

The patron/sage took one breath and exhaled the following words of absolute wisdom: "The work will never be done. There will always be vegetables to wash, soil to weed, and dishes to put away. You will learn that these tasks aren't 'yours' to complete. You have done your part for the time allotted. The afternoon team will take over. Turn off the water and come up to the house now... It's time for lunch."

Mic drop.

And ouch.

Humbling. Humbling to realize I'd be sowing seeds to plants I'd never harvest. And despite my hours, my sweat, and my earnest dedication, I didn't get to call the ends mine. Truly, a commitment to process over product. And letting go of my unyielding, *I-did-that grip*, in place of mindfully doing it, for however long I had.

Do your work, then step back.

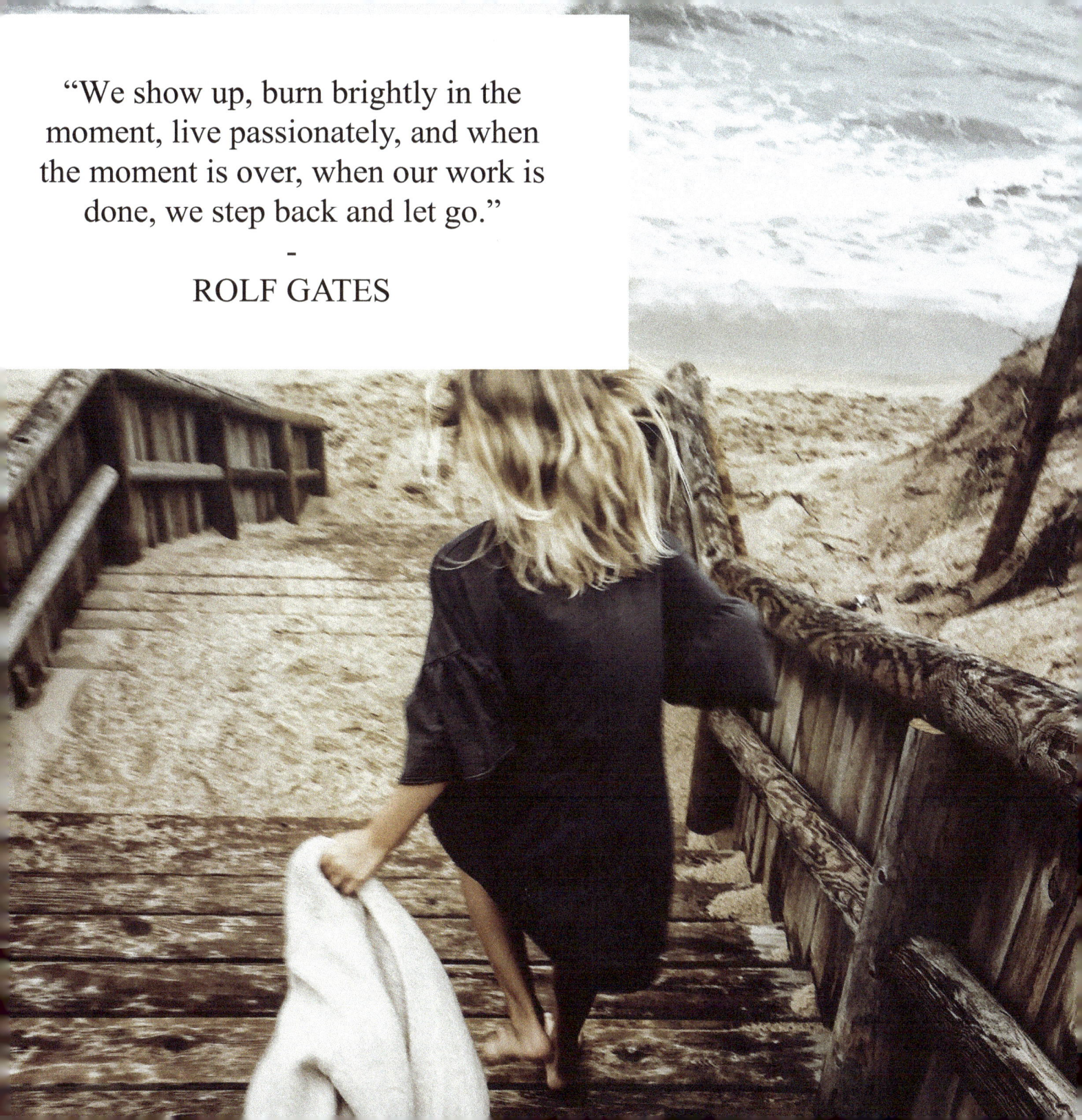

"We show up, burn brightly in the moment, live passionately, and when the moment is over, when our work is done, we step back and let go."

-

ROLF GATES

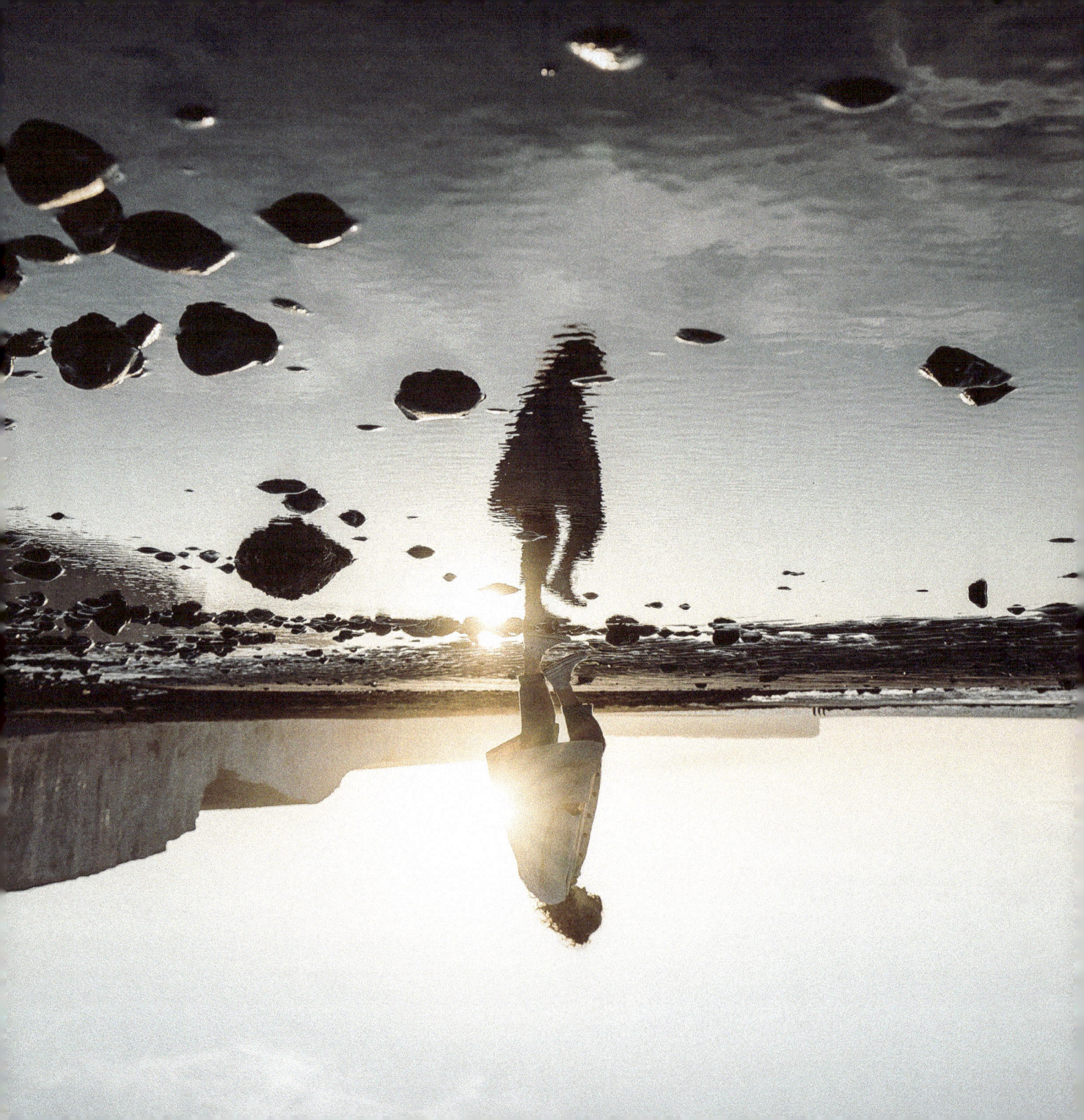

"Meditation is not evasion;
it is a serene encounter with reality."

-

THICH NHAT HANH

Though such a statement is wholly unnecessary in pro-meditator circles, it speaks directly to the meditation-curious. If you are one such individual, you may be thinking "Did this monk just read my mind?"

When we are in the beginning stages of meditation, it is enough to simply be able to sit still for five to fifteen minutes and focus on the breath. As the seated posture and the focused attention become more easeful with repetition, we begin to peel back the layers and deepen our practice. There are indeed oceans and, really, galaxies upon galaxies under the surface if you are open and receptive and wanting to find more.

Above and beyond the life-changing ability to find calm, concentration and awareness, a bit further in there lay the profound understandings about the nature of reality and consciousness and our place within these. No big deal.

For those who have ever thought: "Isn't meditation just another form of distraction? Another way of escaping the stressors of everyday life in front of us—just as a drug, excessive alcohol or some other coping mechanism might do?" Take heed. It is, instead, an "encounter with reality"... truly, the opposite of an escape or evasion. And one that offers us serenity in the process, as TNH here so beautifully states.

For when we meditate and peel back the aforementioned layers of what looks to us like brick-and-mortar REAL, we discover an entirely novel, entirely disguised, Truth. And as this process unfolds over time and with consistent practice, we begin a simultaneous learning and unlearning of all that we thought we knew to be real.

And, if I may be so bold as to join voices with the prolific Hanh, we, in fact, evade every day that we do not meditate. Whether or not you are yet ready for this serene encounter is up to you.

It's a matter of when.

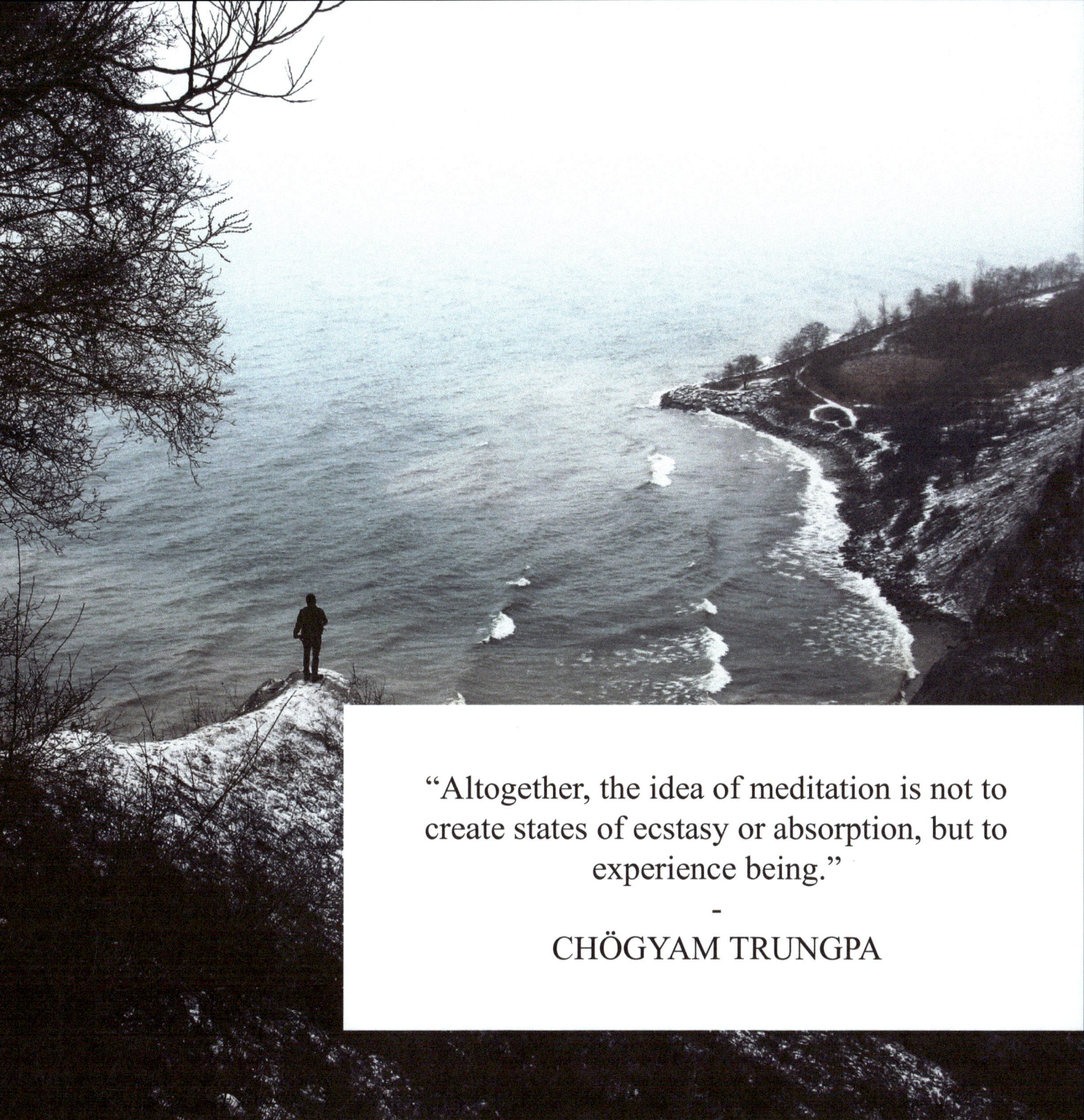

"Altogether, the idea of meditation is not to create states of ecstasy or absorption, but to experience being."

-

CHÖGYAM TRUNGPA

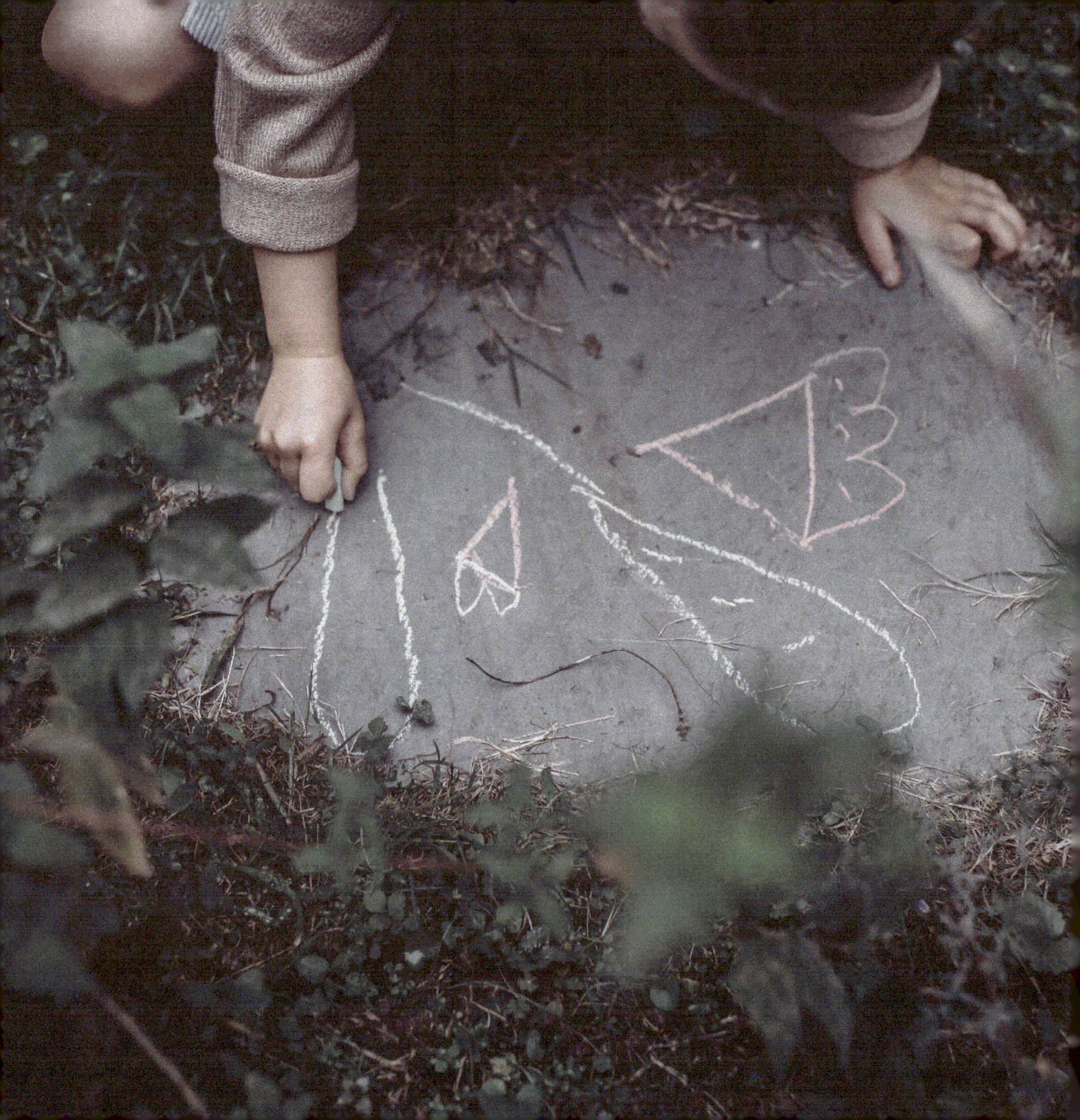

"The mind is everything.
What you think you become."
-
UNKNOWN

Read that again. What you think, you become.

We find the very same notion in the Old Testament's Book of Proverbs, "As a man thinketh, so is he" (23:7). This is also the central tenet in much more recent books like The Secret and in the New Thought philosophy The Law of Attraction. As it turns out, this compelling idea is quite accurate from a scientific perspective.

We know that the brain is plastic. We know we can learn new skills, create new memories and rewire our neural networks toward changed reactions, thoughts, and behaviors, for better or for worse.

The study of Experience-Dependent Neuroplasticity specifically looks at how the brain changes, in structure as well as in function, in response to various experiences. It involves looking at events and exposures across a lifespan and understanding how certain factors (developmental stage, repetition of stimuli, exposure types/lengths, etc.) work to collectively boost resilience or heighten risk in that individual. In short, EDN looks at the brain's capacity for change based on the life lived by that particular cerebrum.

Although the groundwork circuitry is established in early development thanks to genetics, as we live and experience life differently, so various areas of our brains wire, wither and grow differently. [See "Rumination" in the Language section of this book to understand how thoughts that fire together, wire together.]

Here's the key: when we recognize that thoughts are events of the mind, we can begin to understand that what we think and keep thinking—about ourselves, about the world around us, about the limits of what's possible—physiologically changes us. And by altering that so vital part of our central nervous system at every step of our life experience, we, too, mind-body-spirit, are changed.

Who do you want to become?

Try reverse engineering that one.

"If you begin to understand what you are without trying to change it, then what you are undergoes a transformation."
-
JIDDU KRISHNAMURTI

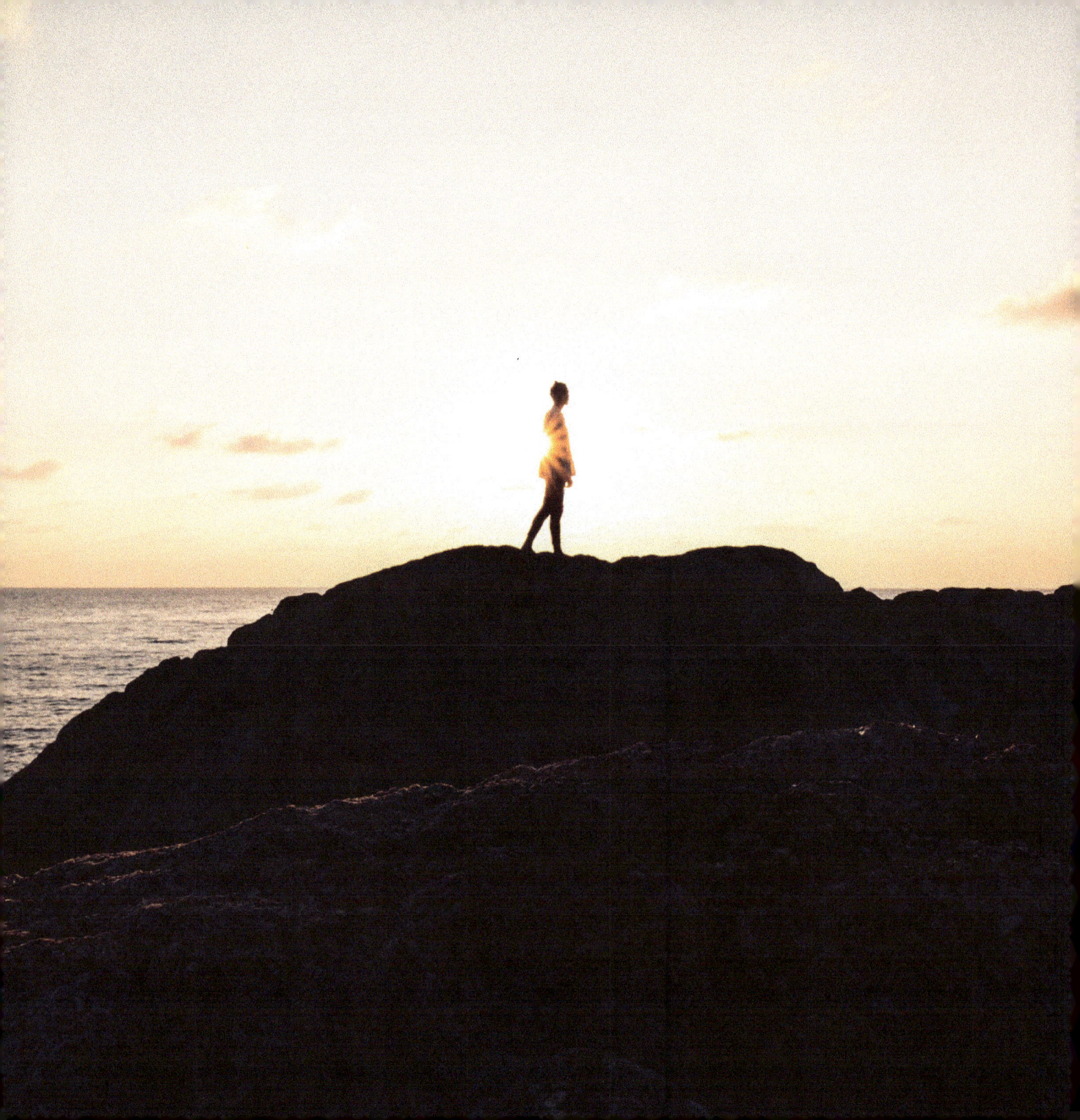

"Peace comes from within.
Do not seek it without."

-

UNKNOWN

Peace.

Isn't this what we're all searching for?

We just want life to feel calm, whole, and joyful without racing everywhere clocking miles per minute. We want to establish, grow, and strengthen connections without these overwhelming our every free moment. We want to lie in bed after a long and wonderful day, feeling grateful, present, and primed for sleep.

Although we may think we are not seeking false idols—that our family is number one and our alignment and priorities are pin straight—it may well be worth taking a moment to truly take stock.

When something in our day goes awry, what *fix* do we seek? Is it coffee or cocktail or (most insidiously) *distraction* with which we medicate? For how many minutes or (gasp) hours a week does YouTube, Netflix, Crave, Pinterest, Facebook, and endless Instagram scrolling hold hands with us, at times so tightly, so unconsciously, we sense it's, maybe, possibly, a bit too much?

And before you think anyone is judging you, recognize that the neighbor to your left and the one to your right are indeed doing what you are doing, at different times and in different degrees perhaps, but one certain thing is that you, friend, are not alone.

Overwhelm and anxiety have become so incredibly pervasive (here in North America at least, though I cannot imagine we are unique) that the demand for so called "innocuous" entertainment has dictated the massive supply.

Enter distraction in the form of (numbing?) fun in every which way imaginable. We could frankly go on for lifetimes consuming, ad libitum. And yet, after all the self-soothing, are we any closer to peace?

Peace comes only from within. I'm going to step right out to the edge of the limb to announce in my loudest, most obnoxious voice: it doesn't come from your work or your passion project, it doesn't come from your podcasts or books… heck, it doesn't even come from your partner or your blessed kids. It's in an untended space inside you.

Even when we *think* we know where to place our greatest attention, unless it's nestling into the cozy center of our consciousness, we've simply missed.

Stop reaching for your phone at the first hint of discomfort. It's more than illusory peace, it's interference.

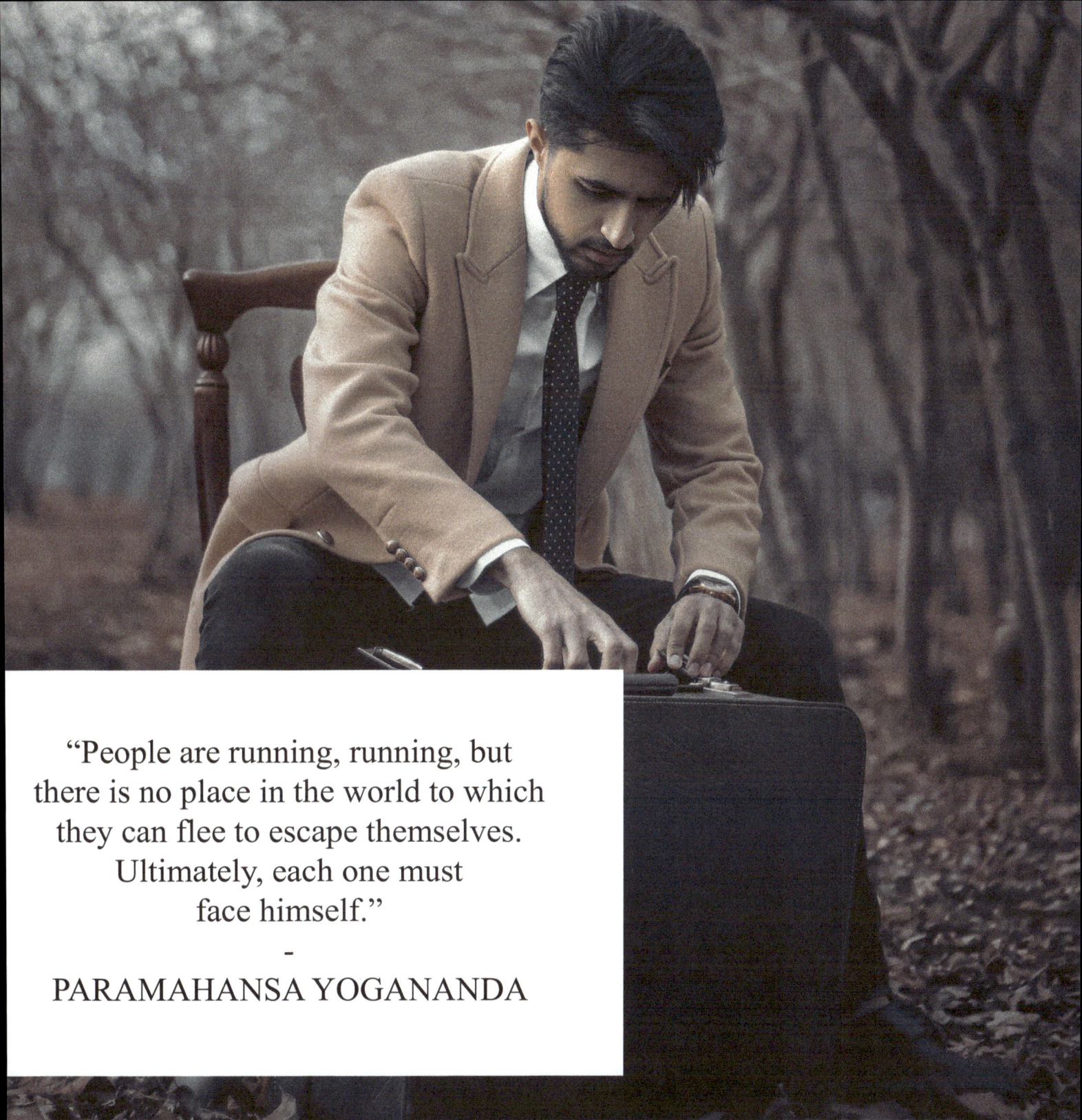

"People are running, running, but there is no place in the world to which they can flee to escape themselves. Ultimately, each one must face himself."

-

PARAMAHANSA YOGANANDA

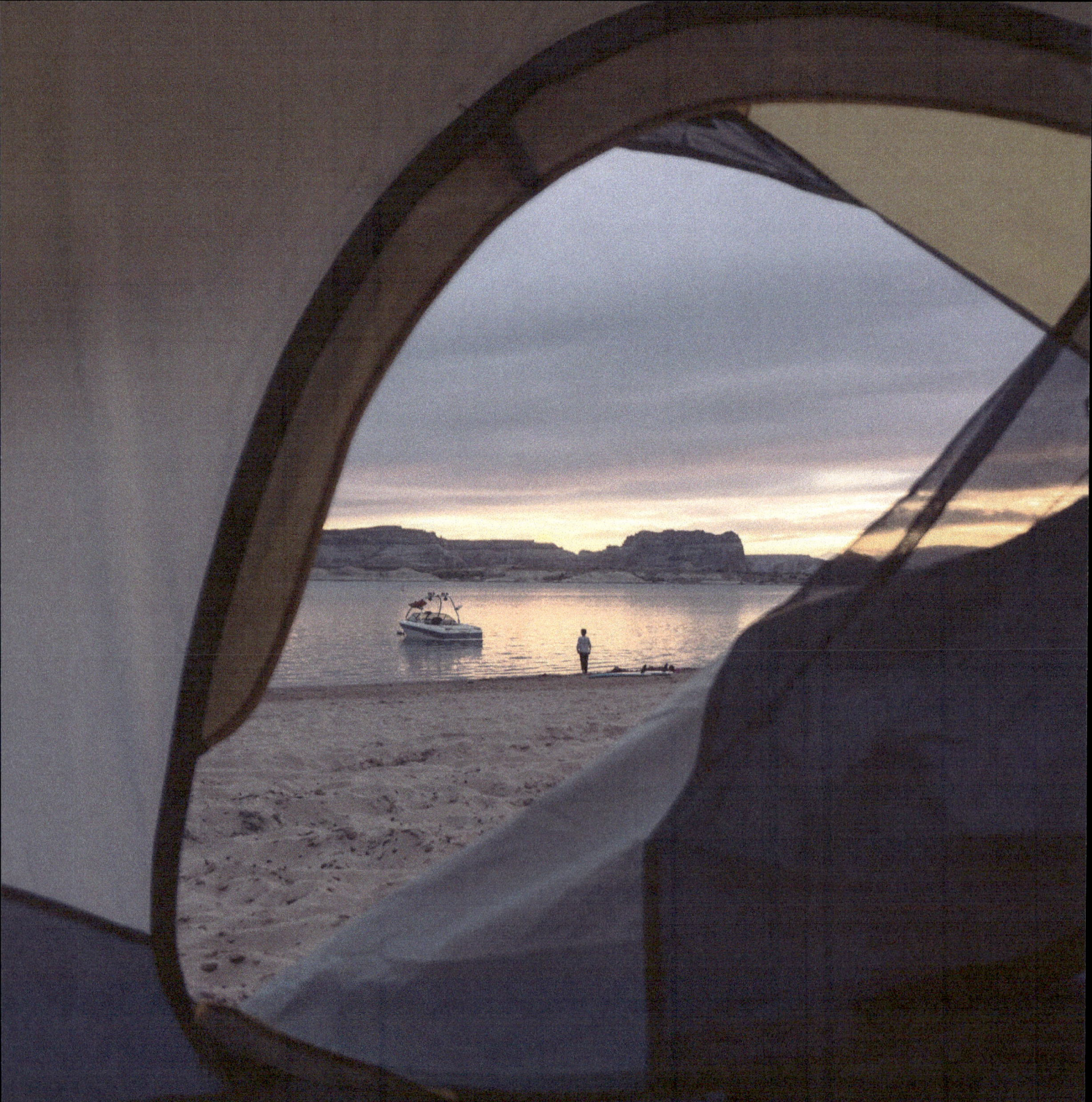

"That's life: Starting over,
one breath at a time."
-
SHARON SALZBERG

Truer words were never spoken.

In its more literal read, we are reminded of that forgotten and for-granted breath. How it truly is responsible for the continuance and maintenance of life itself. I mean, we know this, rationally, but it's an understanding that should, by all accounts, have us bowing down to it about twenty times a minute. Alas, this we do not do.

Read contextually, it is about how mindfulness saves and rebirths us at every moment we remember to remember what's here and now. If we cannot bring attention to this moment and if we cannot wake to the realization that the present is a wholly new moment, then we are doomed to drown in yesterday's pond.

One of the most poignant lessons I've learned through yoga has been the message to let go of all things past. We can do this in the context of a meditation or while practicing mindfulness or yoga. Eventually, we can do this while walking around, going about life.

It's as simple as this: Right now, choose to unequivocally and all-at-once drop that conversation from last week that's been hovering like a small cloud. Decide to let go of the challenges posed this morning as you were trying to leave the house and it felt the universe was conspiring against you. In the very moment you notice its presence, altogether release the hurt, blame, self-doubt, and fear that's plagued earlier versions of yourself to really choose anew. The truth is that you are a different version of you with every breath that passes *only* if you actively decide to let go.

It is often the simplest, most rational concepts that can change everything for us if/when we actually get them. And not *get them* like, "yep, heard that, makes sense, I got it" but actually ah-ha GETTING IT. In Spanish, we would say *hacerse carne*, meaning to "become flesh." Like to in-corporate the understanding into our physical makeup... that level of grasp.

Begin again. Be again.

With every breath, decidedly reborn.

"Imagine holding on to a hot burning coal. You would not fear letting go of it. In fact, once you noticed that you were holding on, you would probably drop it quickly. But we often do not recognize how we hold on to suffering. It seems to hold on to us. This is our practice: becoming aware of how suffering arises in our mind and of how we become identified with it, and learning to let it go. We learn through simple and direct observation, seeing the process over and over again until we understand."

-

JOSEPH GOLDSTEIN

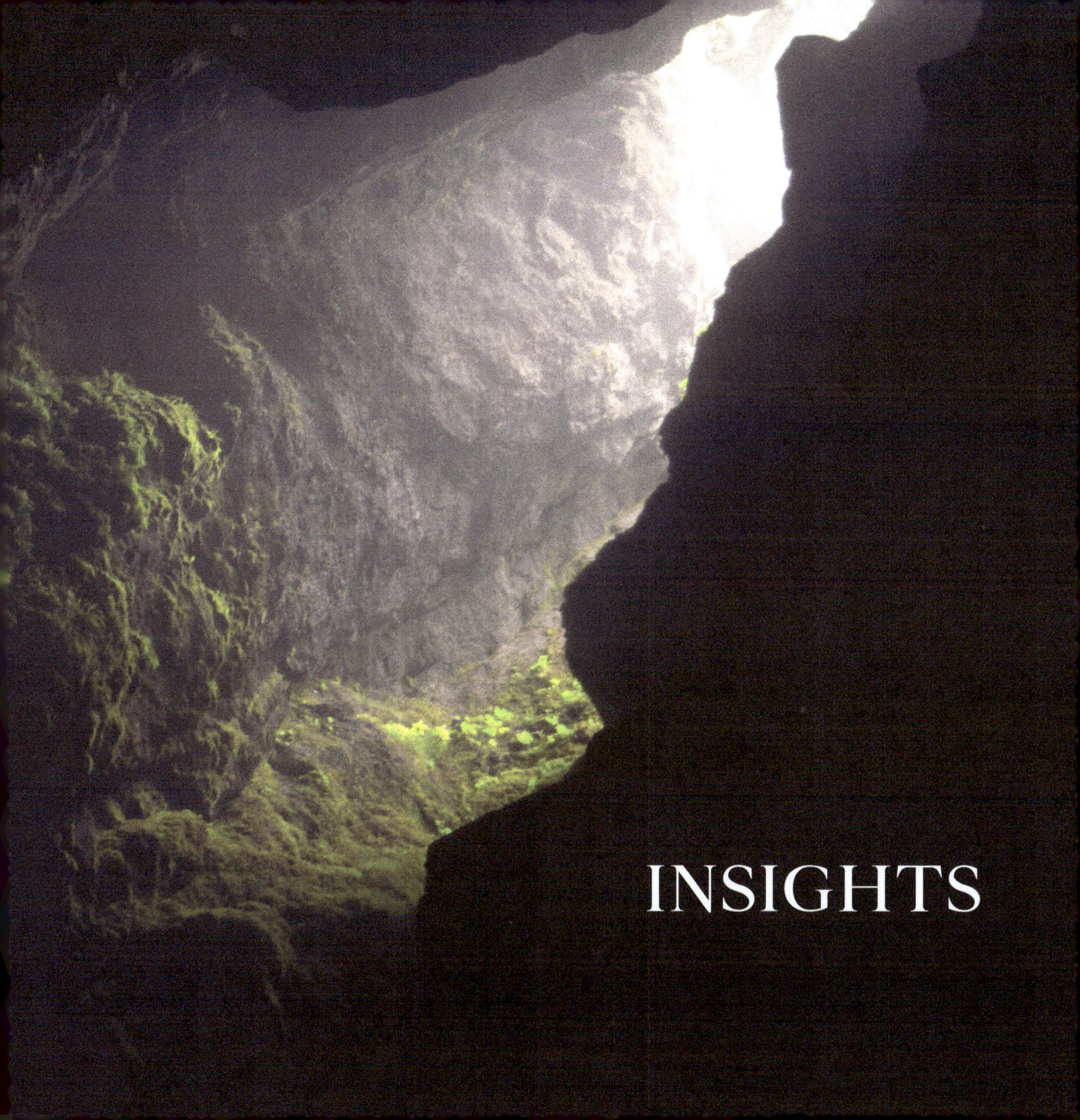

INSIGHTS

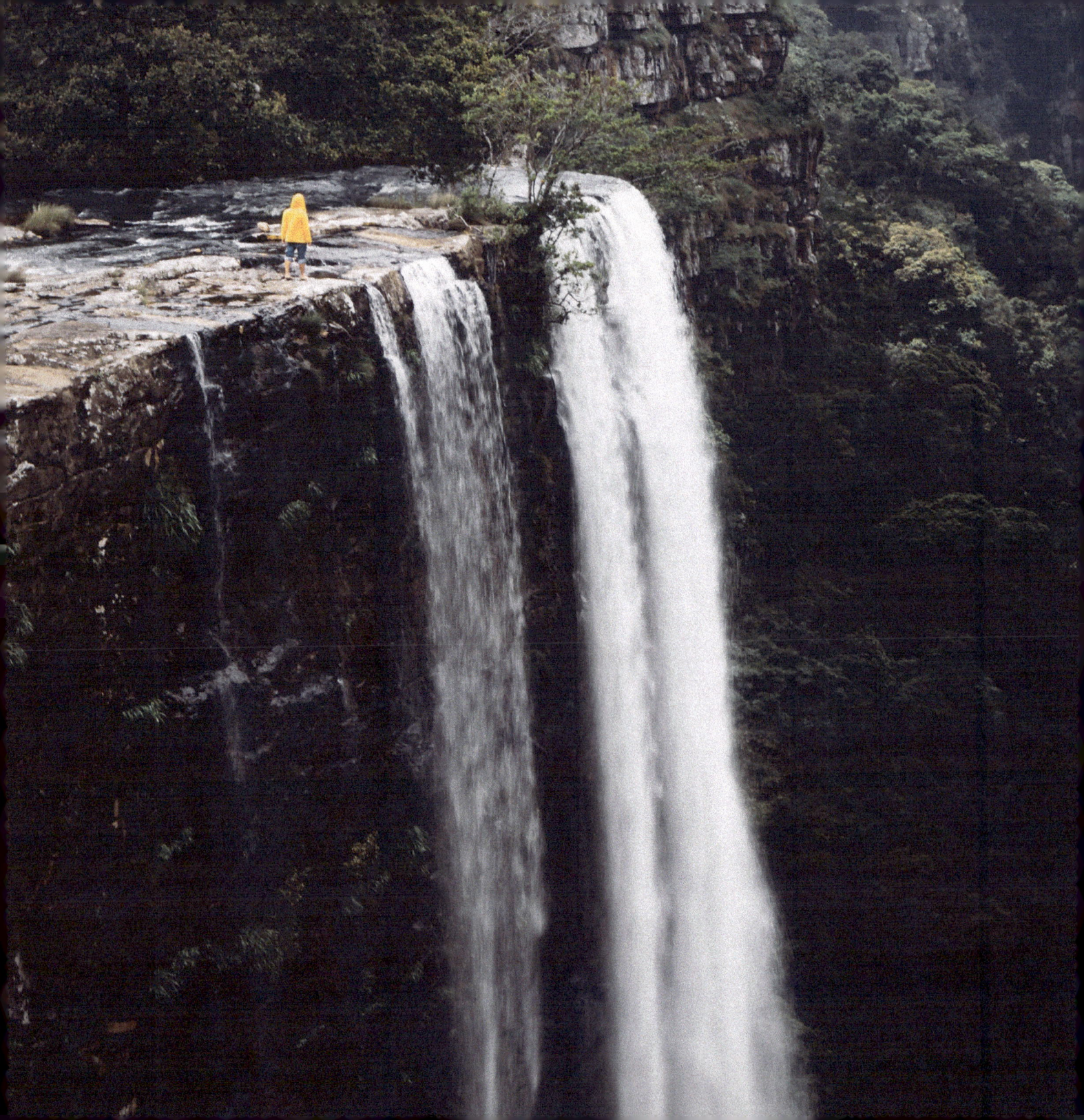

At Your Limits, See What's Real

When we are in onerous times, in those moments that push us to our limits—this is when we can get a clear view of what's really there.

If you have gone through a health crisis, if you have gone through family or professional hardship, you may have noticed that this is where relationships reveal themselves. Where people that you thought would show up didn't, and people that you never would have expected to, really came through. This rings true for friendships, colleagues, family members even.

What drops the veil between *seeming* and *real* is twofold: Firstly, there is a significant perspective shift that occurs in these hard seasons that allows an altogether new view on the things we thought we knew for certain. The who-has-our-back, the what's-really-important, the strengths-and-weaknesses-within.

Secondly, there is what happens without anyone planning or deciding so; niceties and masks and all sorts of things we have no idea we even own (let alone wear) fall away in times of trouble. Almost without our noticing, these cloaks are shed all around us. Crisis in our lives, strangely, calls upon those in our circles to either step toward or to step back. Thankfully, though often painfully, truth surfaces, because to step forward into the space of a neighbor's suffering takes effort. It takes emotional wherewithal, it takes... resources.

Of course, resources are fluid, always relative to a moment in time, to a particular climate or stacking of life-things. Friend x may, at one time, have been better able to support you, but currently is incapable. Cousin y may never have been there for you in the past but, surprisingly, steps up in some unexpected, however welcomed, way on this occasion.

The direction in which someone migrates, then, has everything to do with their *capacity* to be supportive as much as (if not more than) it has to do with their desire or ability to help. Their response, then, does not give us any information regarding the qualitative nature of that particular soul, and one should take care to reserve any such judgement.

Instead, this division—from one row of people in the middle into a nearer and a farther row—helps us find better interpersonal fits, at the very least for that moment in time. The greatest thing we can really take from this reveal is the gift of newly arranged...*equations*, let's call them. Subject-object pairs within our circles that are meaningful on both ends. Where the energetic exchange is fair, accepted and chosen by all parties. A rearrangement of social contracts toward something more genuine.

So, there is some respite when the winds are strong. We really do get what we need.

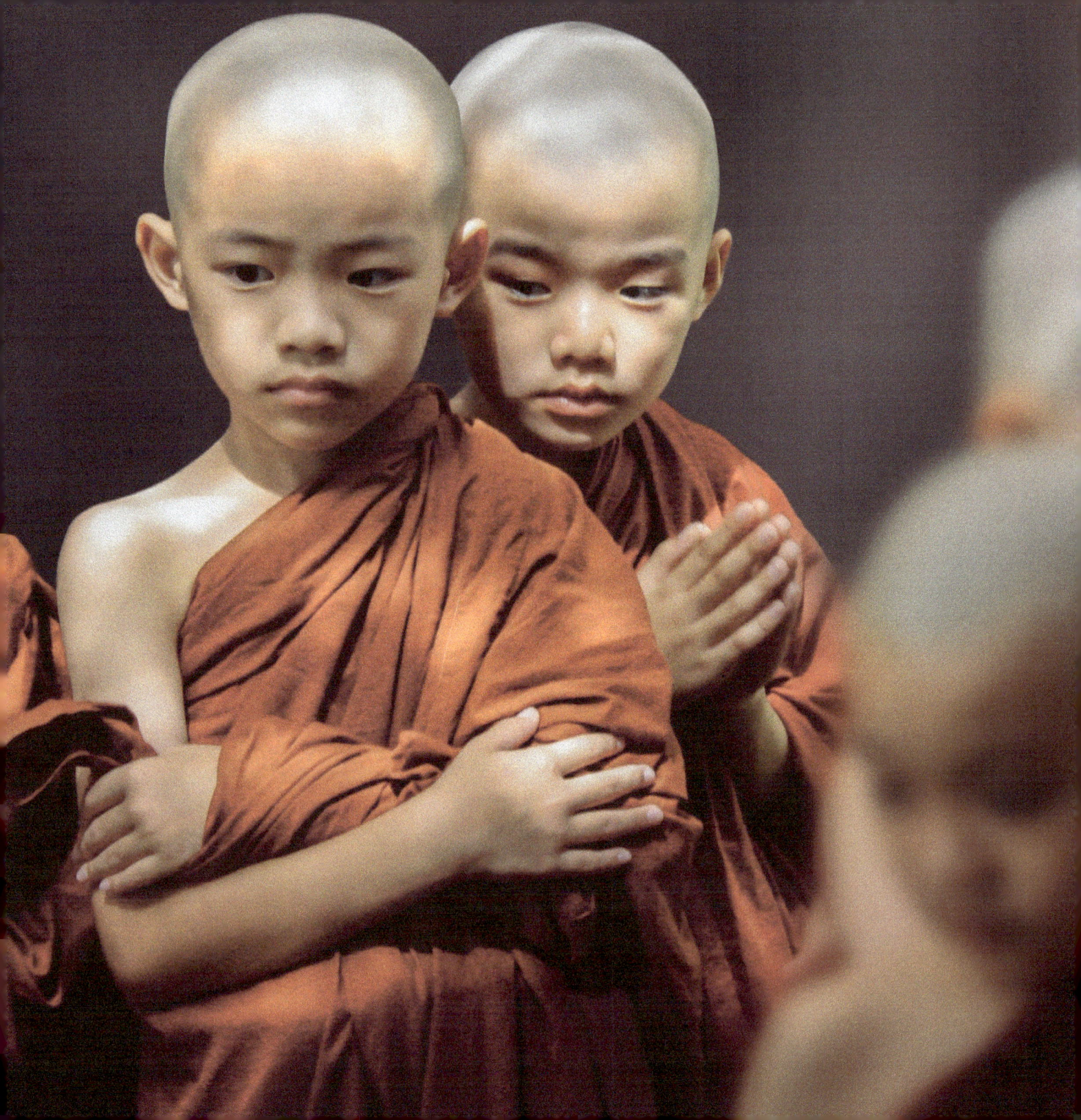

Beginner's Mind

"Umm…nothing's happening. I told you I wasn't good at this."

"It's just the same thing, again and again. I'm not getting anywhere."

"This is boring."

"I've already got that concept, moving on!?"

"Why bother? I've tried this already and I'm not any better."

If you've attempted any kind of breathing, mindfulness or meditative practice on at least a few occasions, you may have had one or more of these thoughts. And often this deters us from coming back to our seat, the very return that will get us anywhere at all.

Where it seems to fall apart is in expectation. Each time we return to the same practice, each time we sit on our cushion or close our eyes, the posture reminds us of what happened the last time we were here. A physical recall. Upon recognition of this set of physical and intentional circumstances, our brains reflexively expect the same thing that happened the time before—and often it's the repeated lack of "thing that happened" that frustrates us even further. Instead of allowing a fresh space, one where anything is possible, we shut down any chance for a different experience. We may also notice that this same thing occurs while away from our proverbial seat; while living our full, layered, beautiful, complicated lives. Do we allow ourselves to awake anew, with everything again possible? Ever?

In the context of meditation, if yesterday I didn't feel anything at all or if a lot of negative thinking came up, if I felt unaccomplished, that tends to be the mind I bring to today's sit. I think: "I know what's going to happen. I'm going to sit, and the same feelings are going to come up. Why am I even doing this? Things aren't getting better", and so on.

Beginner's Mind is a Zen Buddhist concept. It tells us that it doesn't matter where we are in our evolution of practice—of any practice, whether that's yoga or meditation or archery—it doesn't matter at all. If we can hold the mind of a complete novice, we can come to the next seat, the next breath, the next pose, or the next interpersonal encounter, totally fresh. As though we know nothing and have no prior experience, thus no expectation. This simple change in approach does many things.

First off, it creates space. When we don't know what's coming, there is room for anything. Like that first time that you sat down with a new book or in the classroom of a new subject of study. Possibly it was filled with much more excited anticipation. Maybe there was more of a smile on your face than weeks down the line. "I wonder what this is the start of. What might happen? What might I learn?"

The boredom / expectation / premature disappointment doesn't take long to set in.

You may be on day six of a potentially life-long practice, and if you're already thinking you know what's coming, that you know what's possible, the chances of sustaining said practice beyond a few days or weeks are slim to none. I will say this again and again: it is a training. It is like any other course that you would take at school or at work. *It's a training*. It's a repatterning of thought processes. It's a repatterning of behavior, of reaction, and how we view the mind and the concepts of the mind. And the training only works if we train consistently, over time, via repetition. I can forget about becoming skilled in karate if I abandon the dojo a few weeks in.

For both the novice *and* the experienced, it's about approaching each day and each practice with a mental-emotional blank slate. As though each time, we are saying "I have no idea. I have no expectation. And I really have no knowledge." Now, today's practice allows everything in. All is possible once again, and the initial excited anticipation is restored. It's limitless. The page is empty, open. We sense a smile materialize with each and every return. Beginner's Mind is a practice in and of itself, which even Buddhist monks use to further the fruits of their dedication. Thus, we are never expert. We never reach peak skill nor accomplished mastery over anything. Three thousand times in tree pose or none, *this pose right now* is something altogether new. We are lifelong learners, always beginning again.

What if we brought a Beginners' Mind to every conversation with a loved one? Maybe these are the same conversations that we've been having over and over. Maybe they are particularly filled with conflict or are prone to conflict. If there is no prior experience, if we don't think we already know what the other person is going to say or how they are going to react, how differently might that interaction play out?

What if we approached charged exchanges with our children in the same way? Burdensome tasks at work, detested cleaning duties, anything at all?

With a blank canvas, what could be in store?

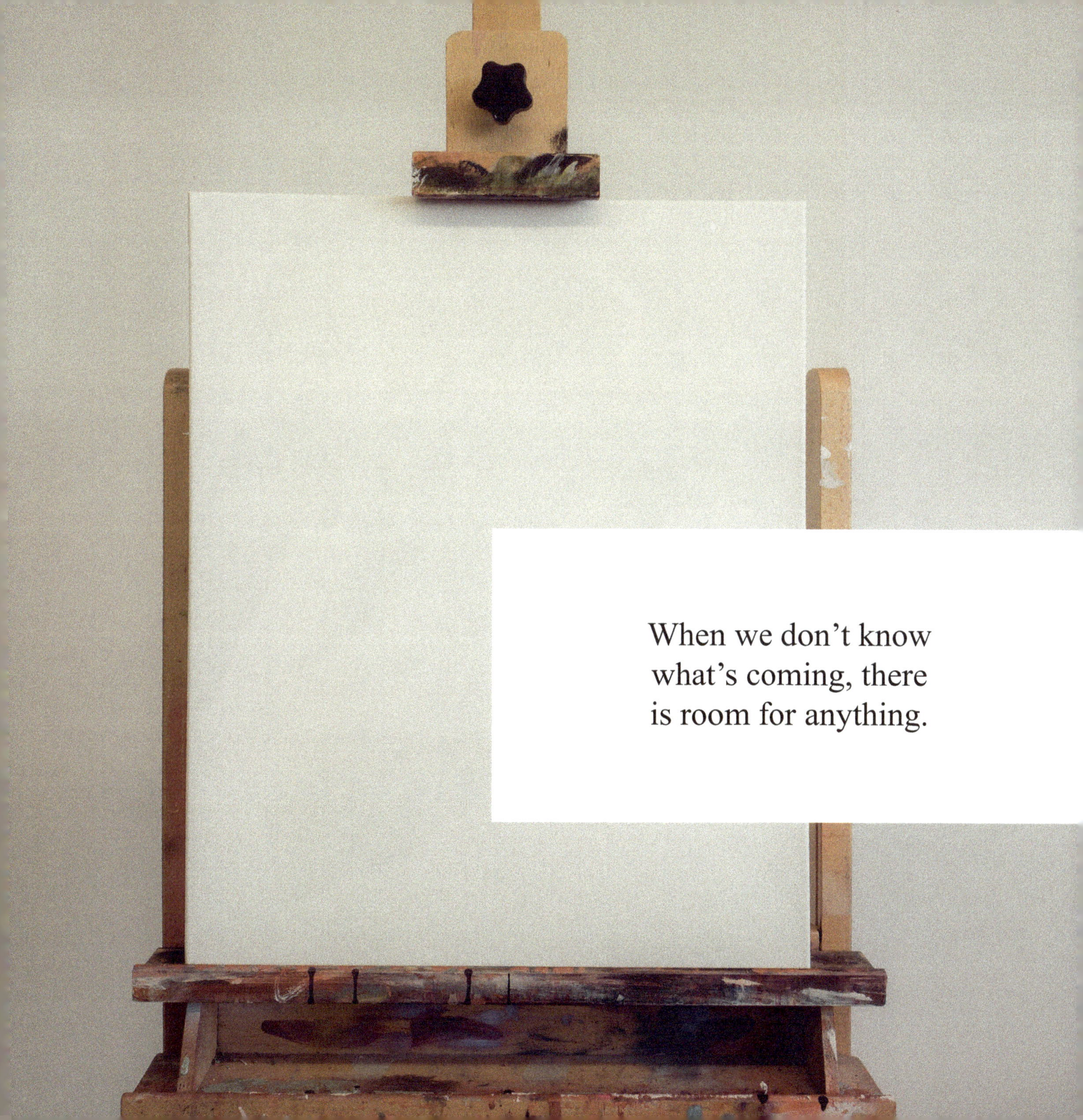

When we don't know
what's coming, there
is room for anything.

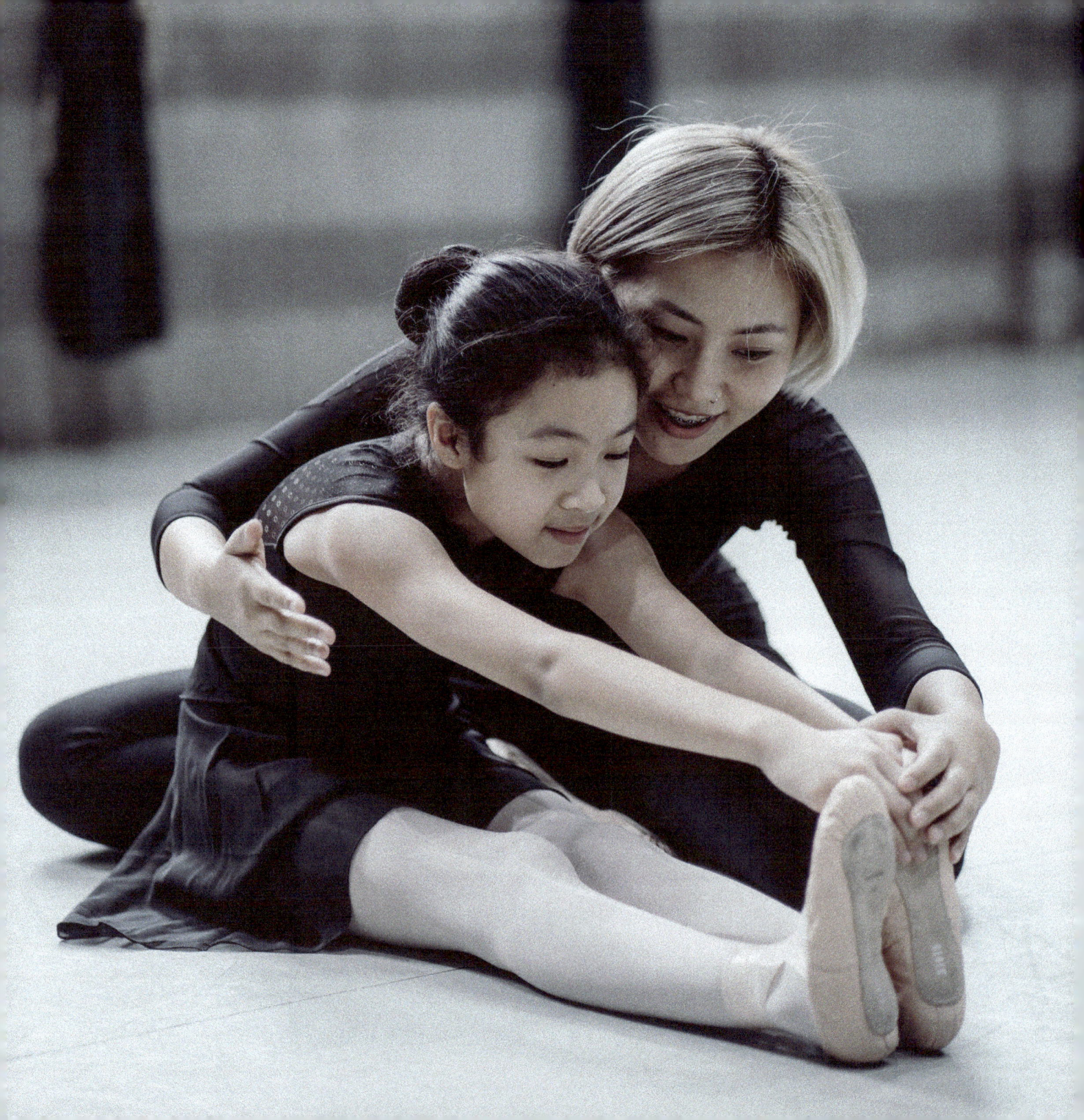

Being Teachable

This is a key aspect of any mindfulness practice that goes hand-in-hand with the concept of Beginner's Mind.

I do a lot of at-home yoga. One day, for some reason, I felt drawn to venture out a bit from my usual classes. I felt explorative. I didn't do any in-depth research. I chose something YouTube suggested and pressed 'Play'. Immediately, in the first minutes of class, I found myself judging the teacher. Ridiculous, completely unfounded, silly human stuff. I had never seen her before. I didn't know anything about her. I thought, *I'm not sure what I'm going to learn here.*

By some stroke of accidental genius (read: by sheer inertia), I practiced on. Probably about halfway through, there appears a pose that I've never seen before in my life. Thirteen-plus years of in-depth yoga study/practice, and I've never seen this before. A surprise, to say the least. All at once, all of my preconceived (admittedly ignorant) notions fell away as though in a waterfall. *Wait a minute. Maybe I'm learning something. Maybe I have no idea what this person actually knows.*

Humbling. Ego-stripping.
All the good medicine.

Thank you, with arms outstretched, to that yoga teacher. Thank you to every experience, every soul that I cross paths with, for the infinite lessons. My ears and eyes are open. I'm here to learn.

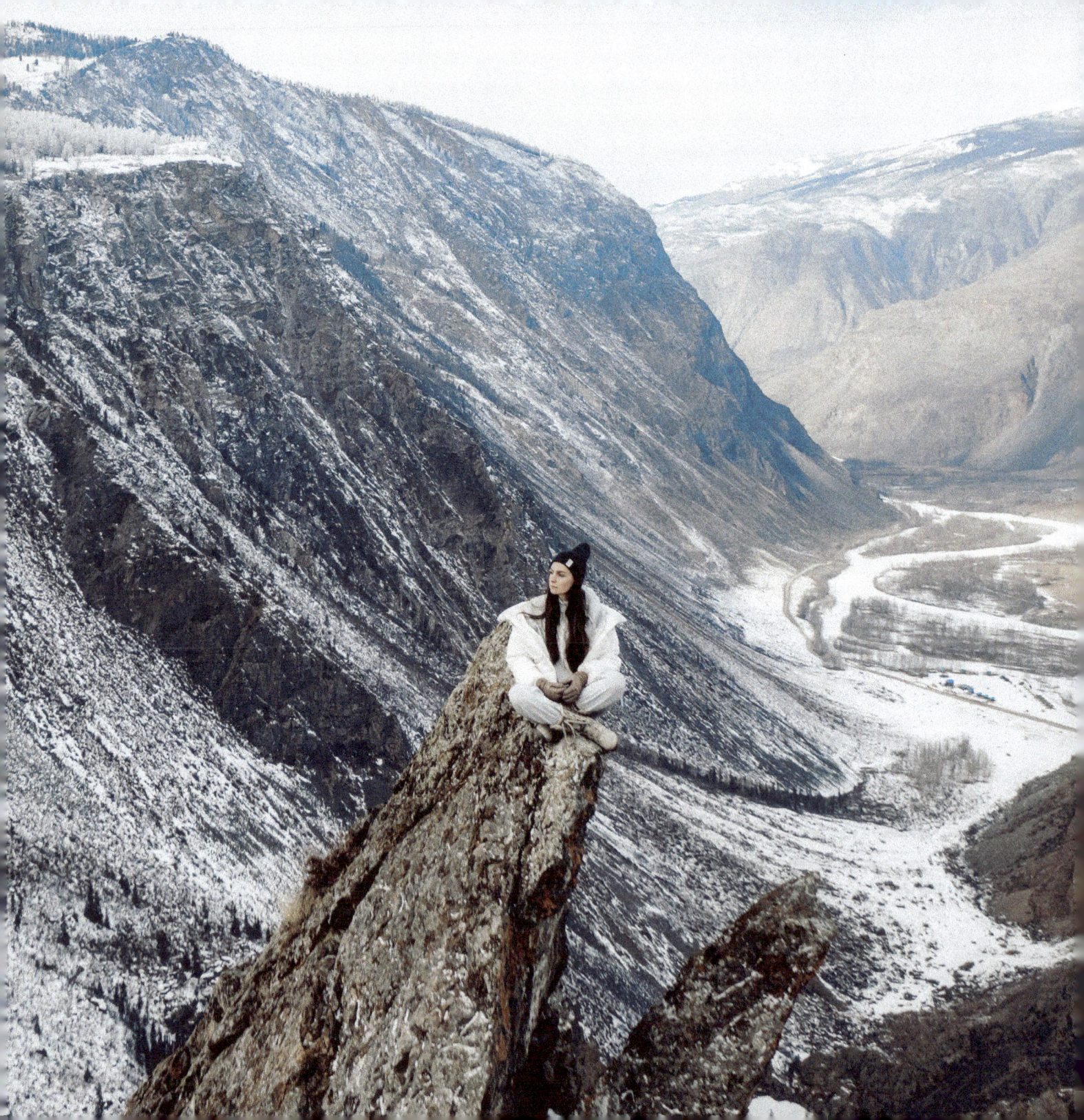

Comfortable Discomfort

Sthiram Sukham Asanam.

Ever heard this phrase? In the context of a yoga class, possibly. Otherwise, not likely.

This is taken from the (great sage) Patanjali's Yoga Sutras written two thousand years ago. Its translations vary, but roughly, *Sthiram* means rigidity, firmness, hardness. It's also interpreted as steadiness or stability. *Sukham* is a sweetness, a peacefulness, a comfort, an ease. *Asanam* refers to a posture, the physical state of being some-where, somehow. Its literal translation is really "seat." In short, the ultimate purpose of all asana (all physical yogic poses) is to hold a comfortable and steady seat.

Sthiram/sukham is akin to the Traditional Chinese Medi-cine concept of yin/yang. In TCM, neither yin nor yang is to be favored; rather, optimal health is equated to keep-ing both in true balance. In working toward whole person wellness, we must attempt to hold equal amounts of the two ends of any spectrum. When the slider moves too far in either direction, we are reliably moving toward disorder and dysfunction.

In the context of a yoga pose, we simultaneously need certain aspects of the mind-body to be firm and stable, while at the same time finding easeful breath, peace of mind, a felt satisfaction. The clearest and most simple way I've heard it described is as a 'sweet discomfort'. The pose should neither be so far toward *sukham* that you aren't doing any of the work, nor should it lie so far the other way, toward *sthiram*, that the struggle negates any possible benefit.

So, to do the work, we need the effort whilst tapping into ease. We need to be able to hold all of the teacher's plentiful instructions without becoming overwhelmed. At the same time, we must remember that a pose can be sweat-and-shake inducing and yet feel quite luxurious and joyful. Since most of us tend toward the hard-effort side of things, the in-class reminders are almost always toward remembering that sweet *sukham*.

Hold those twenty directives, yes, but find your breath. See if you can breathe with ease. Can you relax your shoul-ders, your tongue, your jaw, your gaze? What muscles and holding patterns can you let go of that actually aren't re-quired for all of the alignment principles to still stand?

And if we can find the right places where letting go and pleasure are possible, suddenly the pose changes. It feels different than some moments ago. Perhaps we think, *now this is more comfortable, I might be able to hold this for longer*. Most poses are wonderful for a few seconds, and we feel like rock stars when we can achieve that "perfect" alignment for a few (usually held-breath) seconds. But try holding it for a full minute. Note if your mind perceives this as a stressor.

In my last week at the Sivananda ashram in India, during my teacher training, our instructors asked us to complete the entire class sequence holding each pose for six *long* minutes. Six minutes in Bridge. Six minutes in Headstand. Six minutes in Crow. It's in those moments when we need to go within, to find that ease wherever we can without losing the stability. If not, we simply fall out. Usually, frustratedly.

So here is some real off-the-mat stuff—and this is why I'll be devoted to this practice for the rest of my days:

Those postures, these challenges, they are not *part* of life, they *are* life. In body, mind, and soul, we move from pose to pose, every second of every day. The actual make-up of our earthly existence is an unending string of hurdles to walk through (some exciting, some nerve-racking, some neutral and unnoticed). However we wish to take them, the rolling hills are, in fact, a consistent landscape.

So, when we find ourselves in a particularly difficult moment, how can we find this steady ease? This comfortable discomfort? Though most of us have been conditioned to believe that hard things can only be moved through or overcome with our unwavering hardness (where everything has to be strenuous, where there is no room for rest or levity, where it's all just too much to take), we fail to recognize that ease and breath and calm—and yes, even pleasure—exist underneath all of that muck and mire.

In fact, *sukham* is always already there.

Please note, I am being purposeful with my choice of words. I'm not asking you to *add* an element of comfort or of ease. That's almost more work. What I'm proposing is that we remember what's already there by removing the shroud. Letting go of the story behind Woe Is Me. Accepting and embracing the seeming incongruence of holding both positions at the same time. We can have pleasure at the same time as hardship. We can also have ease. Something devastating may be unraveling, and yet laughter may also hold space in that moment.

How might we bring the same intention of sitting in a pose for six whole minutes to whatever particular hill we happen to be walking? What would we need to do to survive it, keeping in mind its longevity and its integrity? We may find that we'd need to let go of a few things in order to carry on. And allow a few others.

Sthiram Sukham Asanam. Steady and sweet.

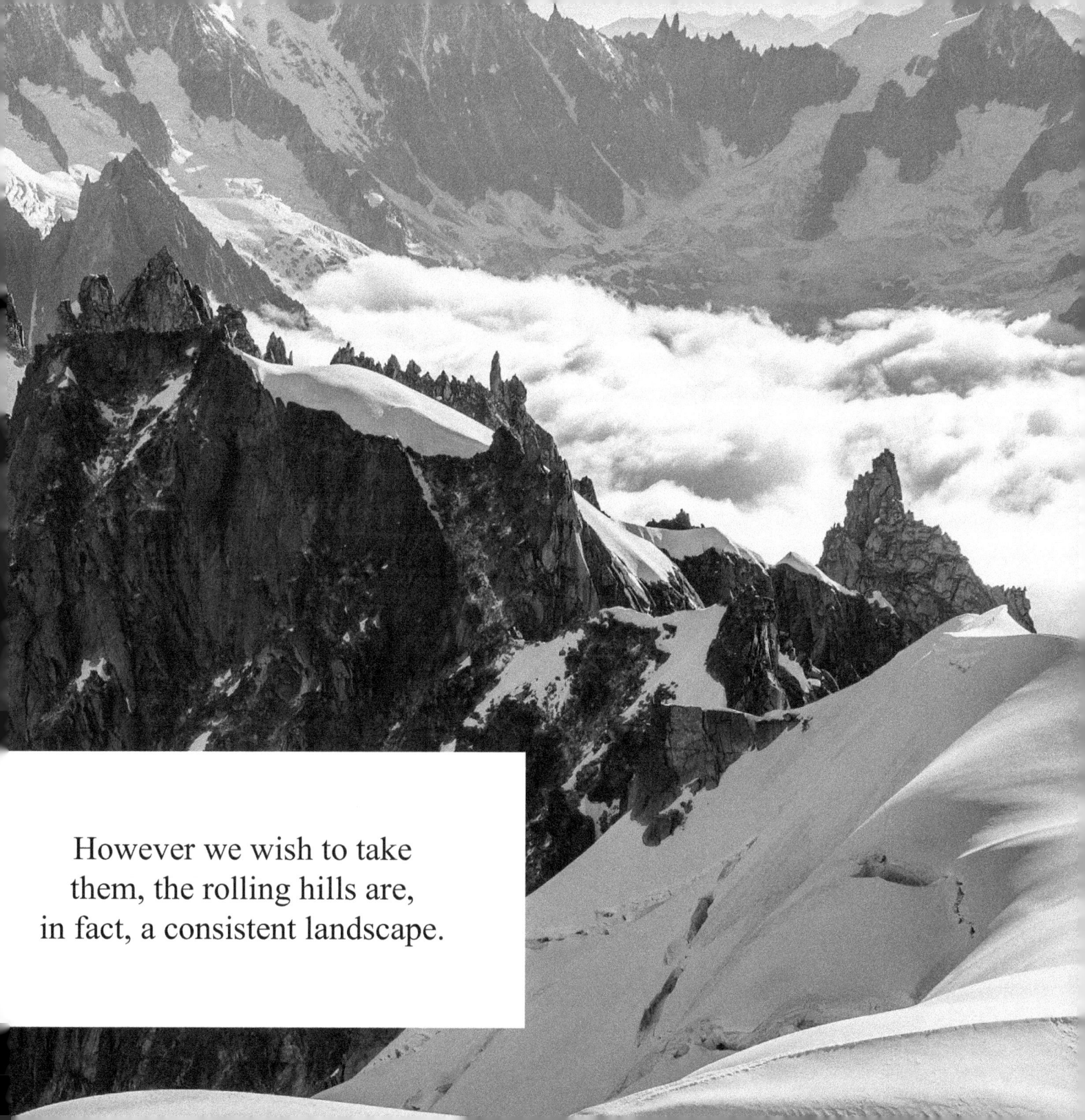

However we wish to take them, the rolling hills are, in fact, a consistent landscape.

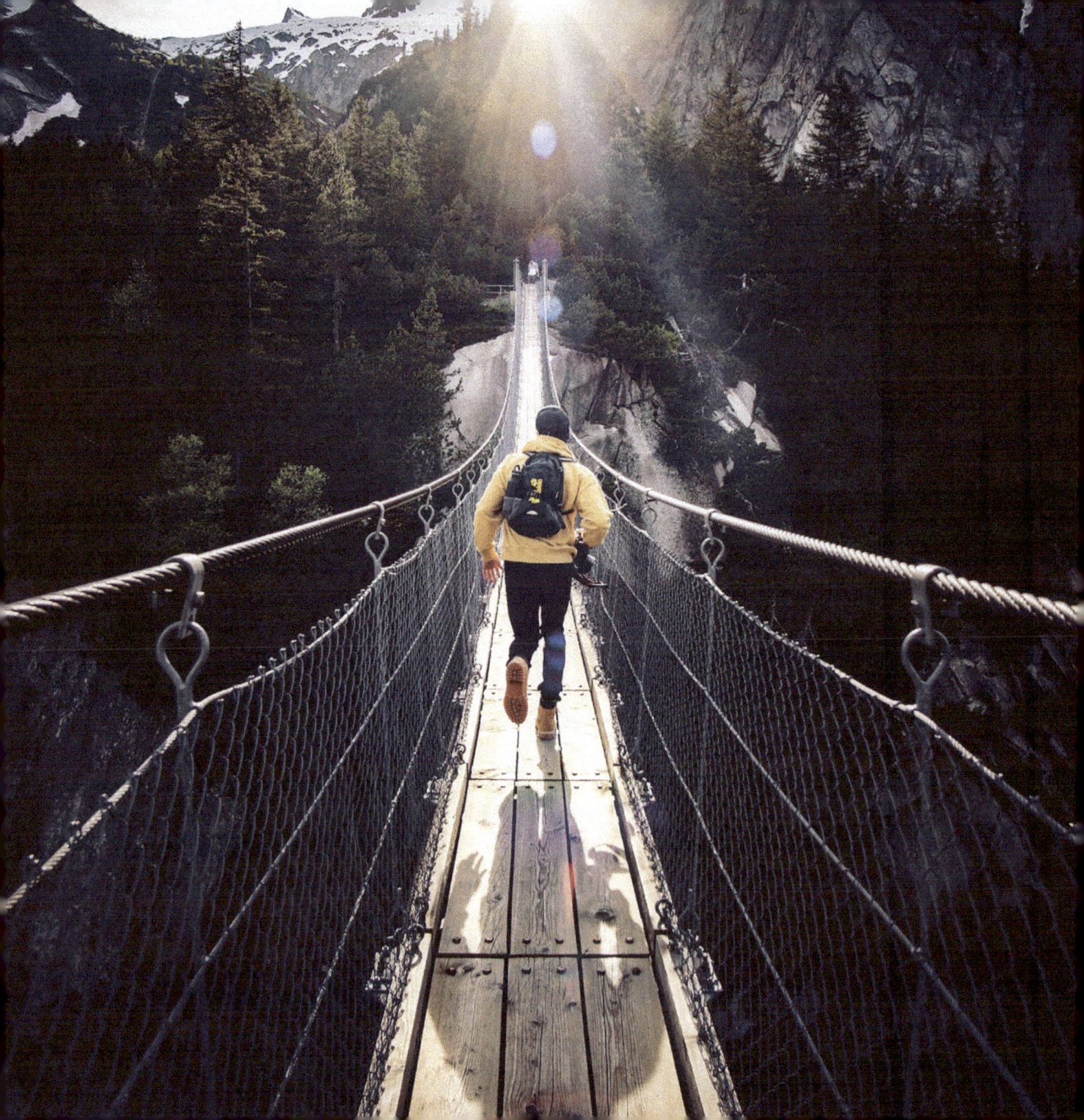

Get Clear

Do you ever feel that things that were once clear in your mind, get…confused? Whether with the passage of time, with having left them on the backburner, having left them unsaid, undone, unresolved? Sometimes those items nag at you to look at them again. It was something that truly needed to be said, that needed to be done and/or that was begging for resolution in your heart or mind, in order to clear the path for something new.

One simple way of regaining that clarity is to move your body. And even more effective is if you can do so outdoors and on your own.

Even if you live in the middle of a suburban desert, try to find even the most minimal green space nearby, some access to a tree or a stream. The on-your-own piece means no babies, no friends, no pets, no phones. And then, you move. Whatever movement makes your body happy: brisk walking, running, cycling, swimming, hiking, dancing or doing back-to-back cartwheels.

The alone part of this is pretty crucial to getting clear. Social movement and group play offer massive benefits of their own accord. But for this specific purpose of regaining clarity, we need time with ourselves. What I'm talking about is getting to a place in that rhythmic breath and movement where you can zone out a little bit.

In any exercise, there is the ever-presence of the body: it wouldn't be exercise if it weren't actively in effort and/or some degree of discomfort. Despite its unending ben-efits, exercise is not all rainbows: It's tough, it's hard work—it's supposed to be. But there's a lot of joy to be found. So, in the midst of that hard work, the body is continually re-minding us of where we are. Getting into our bodies and actually feeling the physical strains and stretches is one of the ways movement actually helps us be here and now. We are too often stuck in our heads, analyzing to overwhelm or anxiety.

So, there is getting into the body. There is also the space *between* body and mind. Runners may talk sprints around getting "in the zone," but let's be real: No matter how avid an athlete you are, it's simply not the case that we outright *forget* that we're exercising. There are moments though. Pockets. Seconds—or if we're lucky, minutes—where distractions and even the body's current efforts fall away from our attention. We zoom out without trying, and zone out. We're in flow. To me, this is the space between.

As the distractions blur and become quiet, the confused items on that back shelf of our consciousness seem to instantly clarify. It is as though the repetitive movement and breath and the letting go of certain held mental patterns run a fresh and forceful gust of of air over the things that need attending.

They are, once again, bright, shiny, completely clear and in view. Time to do this with that situation and put this one in the ground. Time to deal with this thing and let that one go. This happens all on its own. And you can set the intention for where you'd like to direct that gust of air.

Here's a little activity to try: A great yogi once taught me that if I had any lack of clarity or question in my heart, I should pose it to myself just before practice and then let it go. And that, either within that session or within the few that followed, the answer would reveal itself.

When you are outdoors, moving, on your own, you begin to come back to you. You start to get really clear. You re-member things you had forgotten. Promises that you had made yourself or determinations that you had come to that were once meaningful and have since been forgot-ten or put aside. Somewhere along the way, these have been clouded and muddied.

Because life is a bit messy that way. Life is a lot messy that way. How many of us really have the time and space to immediately attend to every potentially important thought or idea that pops into our brain? How often are we able to drop everything, there and then, and say, "Let's work this out," and proceed to journal for hours? (In an al-ternate universe, all of us!)

See what happens when you attempt this intention set-ting within the context of movement outdoors. Think of something unresolved or some unanswered question you would like insight on.

Bring this to mind before you leave the house, and simply see what is revealed. See if you can effortlessly find the space between and get clear.

Entering this space on a repeated, consistent basis, we find ourselves again.

As the distractions blur and become quiet, the confused items on that back shelf of our consciousness seem to instantly clarify.

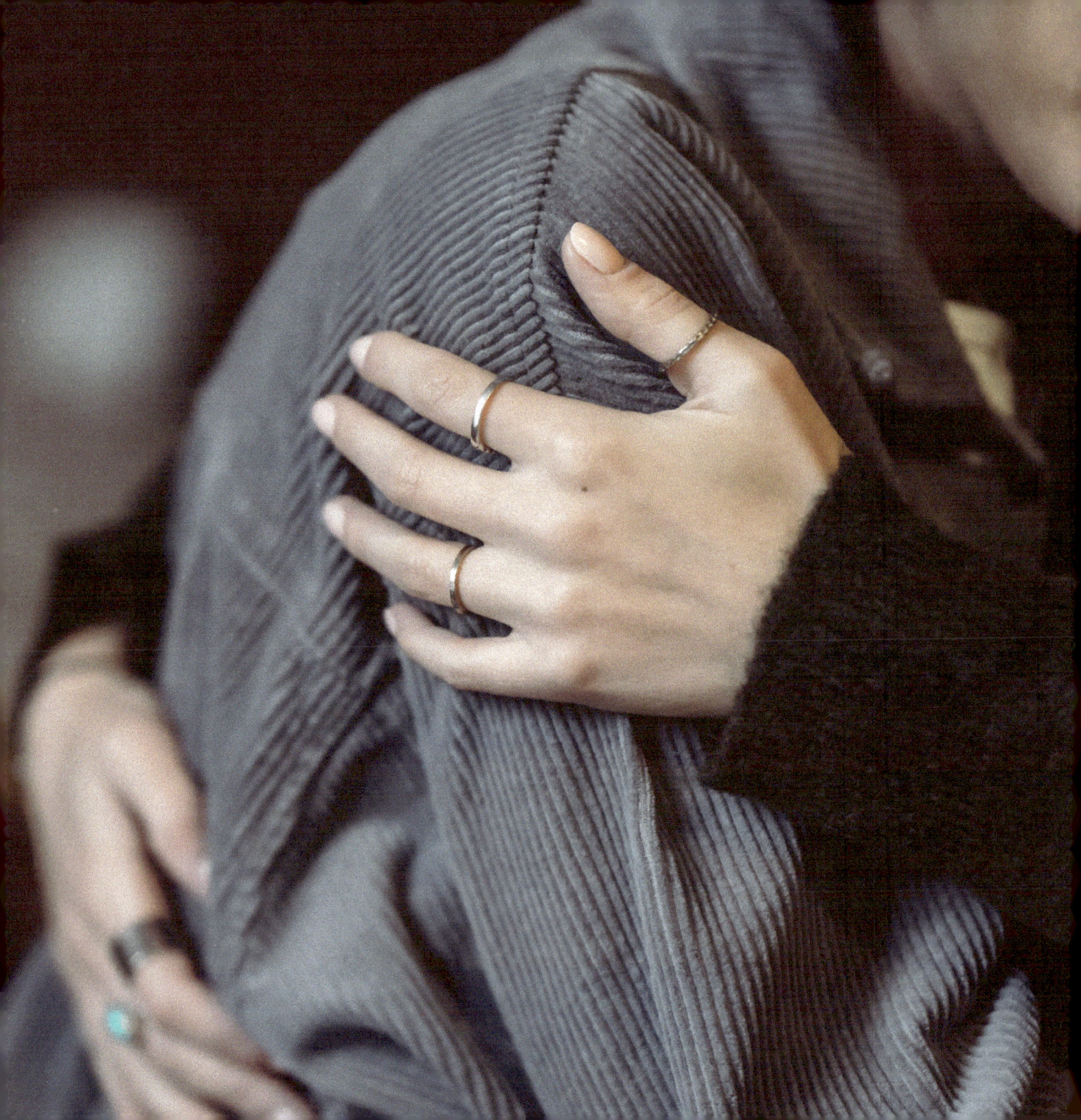

Go Easy

I once read an article about a man who had just lost his father. Mere hours later, this man finds himself in the grocery store, examining a bunch of bananas. In his first-person account, he recalls catching himself in that rather surreal moment thinking, *What am I doing? My father just passed away, and I'm out buying groceries*. It's easy, of course, to understand and empathize with this human in this particular moment. It's autopilot. Certainly, it's the shock speaking when in that moment we hear *Keep moving. Just do something*. What the mind isn't clearly articulating is the confusion that is resulting from a completely unexpected event crashing upon the quotidian. What it would be saying if it were fully conscious in that moment is *I don't understand. I can't comprehend this quite yet. I have no thought-out response*.

The author, in writing his personal account of the moments following his profound loss, had some very simple yet powerful advice for his readers. Two words. "Go easy," he pleaded. We can never quite know what others in the grocery store, at the bank or at work are struggling with at any particular time. We may think we know something about the lives of others, but we have no idea. We are billions of people, walking by one another, carrying many things under the surface. If, at all times, we assumed that every person that crossed our path was in distress of some kind, how would we act differently? Would we treat them with more kindness? Would we be more patient? Would we smile more? Would we offer our support, ask more questions, and truly listen for their answers? Of course, not everyone we interact with will indeed be so acutely struggling in that very moment. But what, pray tell, is the harm in treating them as though they were? It really is a vicious cycle we play into, with each everyday encounter. Somebody's got a scowl on their face, and we're thinking *"You know what? You're miserable. You deserve your mood."* If we just assumed that the root of all scowls or short temperedness or road rage were really significant personal turmoil, we just might go easier. Truly, what the other needs in that moment is the precise opposite of our trigger-fast, unmindful reaction.

Think of a time you really couldn't be bothered to smile for another, when things felt just too overwhelming, too tragic or too hard to put in the effort or to care how others perceived you. What reactions would you have appreciated?

I have vivid memories of my mood being completely changed by a bus driver. On a moody day of my mine, a sweet, life-loving driver offered me a really huge smile and genuine greeting despite my forlorn expression. Though I'm not sure I dropped my pout enough for him to notice, as I walked to the back of the bus, I felt my spirit shift. The unexpected positivity, even from a complete stranger, was everything I needed. Where there is dearth, nourish.

More love. More compassion.

Go easy.

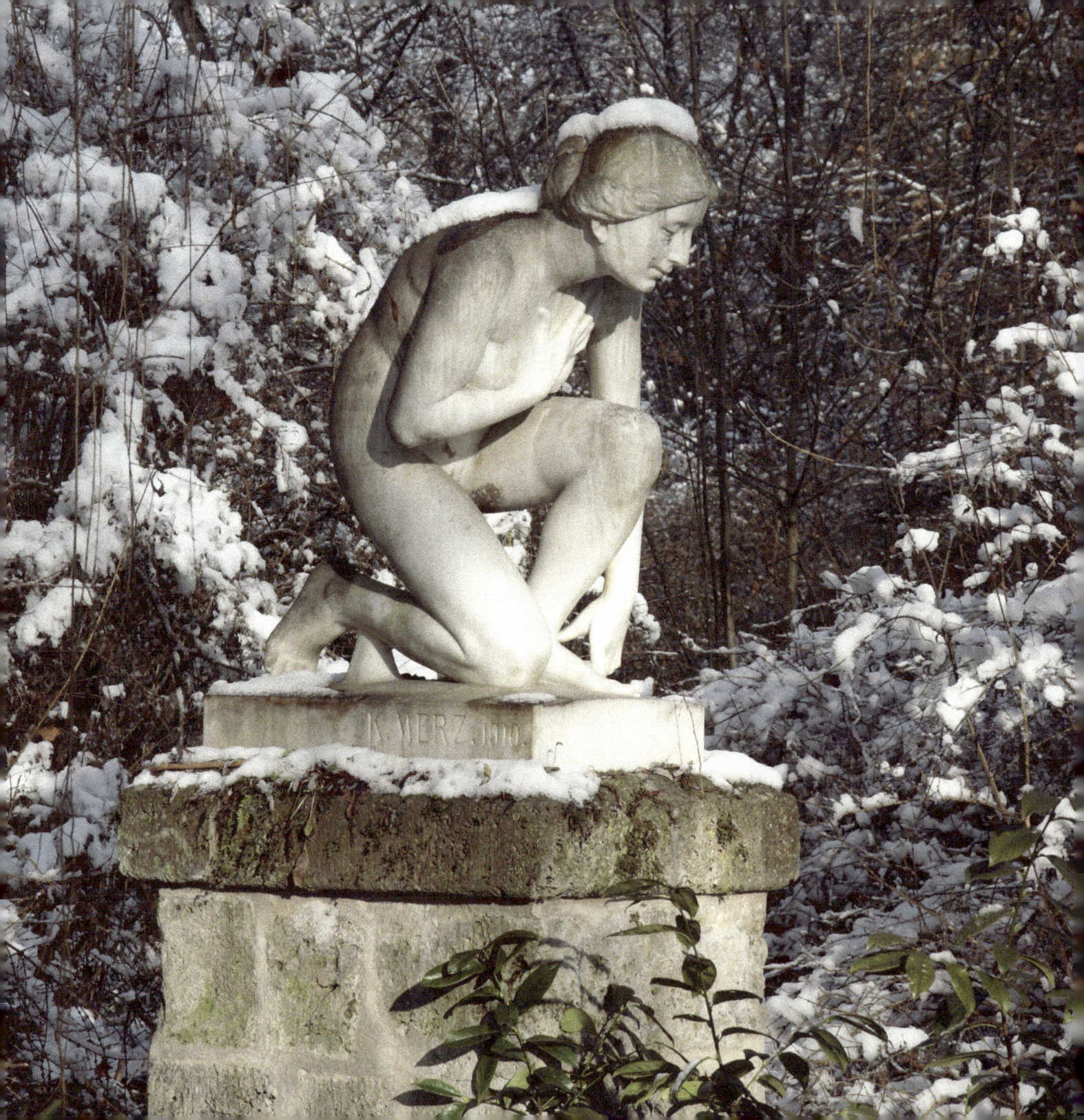

K. MERZ 1910

Living with Heart

What is the true distance between our heads and hearts? Where does that space lie, that space we refer to when we describe acting on feeling, intuition, empathy or kindness? Surely it is not physically within the four-chambered muscular organ lying just beneath and left of the sternum. Surely not there, despite it being the area we place our hands when we attempt to connect with intention, swear an oath, or speak from our truth. As we refer to this physical space as purposely distinct from the brain in our heads (that which is rational, logical), the bundle of nervous-fatty tissue within our skulls certainly cannot be the center of this empathic place, either. Is the 'heart' we mean somewhere in between? Somewhere else entirely?

For a moment, let us offshoot toward a very brief discussion of chakras—the energetic centers within the human body first mentioned in Hindu and Buddhist texts thousands of years ago. Chakras have been understood and described in various ways over the centuries, usually referring to the areas along the spinal column of intersection between many crisscrossing energetic channels. These powerful nodes in the network have been described as central aspects of the "subtle body," meaning all things emotional/spiritual/mental (as distinct from the physical body that we can scan or touch or otherwise measure).

Interestingly, the *ajna* chakra, said to be between the eyebrows or in front of the brain, is also known as the "third eye." The *anahata* chakra, said to be in the center of our chests, is also known as the "heart chakra". You may have heard this referenced in a yoga class when back bending expands the chest in a heart opening pose. Are these focal points of the subtle body the elements we are unknowingly connecting with when we speak of hearts and minds as non-physical concepts?

Wherever they are housed, they can be worthwhile tools in helping us choose attitudes and behaviors in living our lives. A *heart-centred* approach, for example, can prove very helpful in both decision-making as well as in conflict resolution.

To the first point: When making an important decision, where do we find the best answers? Whether it's changing jobs, moving house, deciding to pursue or leave a relationship, or even decisions that aren't quite so outwardly big (but which are personally meaningful for us), what data bank or support space do we run to first? I'd hazard a guess that, for most, it's logic: What makes *sense* for me? This emphasis on logic is a reflection of how much value we tend to place on the thinking brain. What makes financial sense? What is practical, realistic, doable? Which decision has the most checkboxes behind it? This is where your parents will go, this is where your best friend will go, this is where your partner will go.

Because (at least in the North American culture I grew up in), the rational is where we are taught to place stock. It's what follows naturally from valuing IQ over EQ, higher education over life experience, etc.

To be clear, I'm incredibly grateful to have my brain and to be able to use it, trimming and growing connections as I walk the Earth. This is in no way to slight the supercomputer that makes us tick and has me awed daily.

Sometimes, what's rational is precisely that thing that we *should* do. When we feel totally in line with our logic. When we've written out the pro/con list of all the things that do and don't make sense, and a decision that we feel connected to and comfortable with is revealed, by all means, we move forward with it. We've checked in and indeed it's our own decision (not someone else's) and we feel there's no disconnect there? Onward.

Other times, we've made that list and everyone around us, emotionally unattached as they are to the issue, reminds us of the rational thing to do. Our logic agrees. We're in the process of trying to convince ourselves fully. And yet there is something that just isn't clicking. The cogwheels aren't quite fitting... and it's halting the entire process. We feel incapable of moving forward. We are resistant to moving ahead with that decision, despite all the good sense it seems to make.

Here's what I propose for those times: we've got our pro and con list, we've got everybody's opinion, we've got all the things that could be helpful in making this decision. Now we let them go, if for a short while only. Those things

aren't about to disappear, you can even write them down to make sure they can't slip away, if that's helpful.

Take a moment to release it all.

Momentarily move away from all noise: not only outer chatter but that within. Try to consciously slow the pace of our own constant, often exhausting, intellectualization of absolutely everything that we experience.

Now dismantle the rational—not because we should be proceeding with our lives at all irrationally, but as a thought experiment that adds valuable information and somewhat fills the gaps between. *What if I let go of all that logic?* If I didn't pay attention to any of those things that do or don't make sense and just listened to something else? Call it *Heart*. Call it a *Wise Mind* or *Intuition or Gut*. Call it whatever you like. What feelings are there? Does that tabled plan of action feel right, or does it not feel right? Remember, for the purposes of this thought experiment, it doesn't have to make sense.

How often have we heard from an acquaintance or loved one "I'm probably going to take that job, but I really want that other one," or "I don't understand why I think I should be doing *that thing* when it doesn't make any sense to me." If we can sit in that feeling, and if we can figure out that feeling, we've got one new piece of data to inform our decision. And one, I'll argue, that strengthens the reliability of the outcome.

What I want for all of us is to be able to move forward in our choices feeling entirely connected to them, without the natural resistance (and, often, the inevitable future resentment) that presents itself when something *just doesn't feel right.*

So, sit in that heart space. Feel whatever arises. And while it would be foolish to choose our actions based on this alone, bringing some of this heart element into the decision-making process allows us to understand otherwise unspoken resistance, to proceed intelligently and intuitively, with full coherence. No icky, ignored nudges. No unchecked feelings. Just peace.

The other avenue that would benefit from becoming connected with heart is conflict resolution. Think of someone you know, possibly love, with whom getting ideas across is a major struggle. We've all experienced those patterns of communication that aren't really communication at all. They generally consist of speaking, reacting, not feeling heard, reacting back in stronger or louder terms to achieve this...on and on in a vicious cycle.

Two people, with their own ingrained communicatory styles, each deeply connected to their own argument(s) and wanting only for their point of view to be witnessed, acknowledged, and responded to. Yet each party has their own agenda, one that really doesn't include the other, thus they always end up in the exact same place.

How many of us can relate to this? "I know where this is going. We always go here." The item at hand may be different, but the pattern isn't. Left unchecked, we have to understand that the exchange will always go there, and we should be completely unsurprised when, yet again, it does. This is especially true with people that we have a long history with; a parent, a sibling, an old friend. Those relationships where we feel more comfortable in expressing our needs because unconditional love tells us we're safe to do so. While this level of comfort can be a wonderful and empowering thing, it's also true that it allows us to slack a bit in our efforts toward the other party, toward making them feel as understood as we'd like to be.

At what point do we decide to make active efforts against the repeated pattern, in which neither half is satisfied? Here is where we must confront that which we've always done. Standing our ground in the ways we always have simply *has not worked.* This is not to suggest that we let go of the things we feel strongly about or that we drop all attempts to communicate this to our loved (or not so loved) one.

Certainly, though, wanting a different outcome begs a different approach. *Where we can find compassion and love is where we may disarm the other.*

Just imagine the next time that same pattern of communication begins, we recognize it ("here we go again") and we implement mindfulness—we're here, in this place, right now, recognizing the dialogue as something we've seen many times. We acknowledge wanting it to change course and that we are instrumental in that. All of this is an awareness. It happens in a moment. A short pause even in the midst of auto-pilot argument. It might take us many sentences, minutes, or hours, to take a pause and *not* say that next thing that we would always have said before. However long it takes isn't relevant. What's crucial is for it to arise at all. We catch ourselves, at whatever point, and *consider the other*. We consider love and compassion and kindness, no matter how little of this we are currently feeling directed our way.

Some questions to ask ourselves:
- (How) Can I speak more kindly?
- Is there something that this person isn't getting from me (something I might appreciate in turn) that would help them feel heard?
- Can I press pause on my own aims (if for a moment only) to attend to, or at least really listen to, theirs?

Maybe it's as little as silence: letting the other say what they wanted to say without interruption or defenses. Something as simple as, *I acknowledge that that's how you feel. Thanks for letting me know.* Maybe it's a hug or a nod. Maybe it's as simple and genuine as saying *I really don't want conflict with you. How can we do this differently?*

Although effective communication really does require

both parties to be willing, it's almost always true that both won't come to this conclusion at the same time. One will always have to make the first step in breaking such a long-standing cycle.

It is useful, I think, to consider the quality and quantity of our response in this way: the more negativity directed towards us, the more compassion we're being called upon to offer. In that moment, especially in that moment, this is much harder work than continuing the reactionary argument-as-usual. It's an uphill hike and doesn't immediately satisfy any of our own needs. But giving more here doesn't mean giving in. We have to be able to distinguish these things.

We learn to recognize resistance, offense, and conflict and we get used to responding with equal but opposite forces. So, *to your hurtful comment, I will tell you I'm sorry you are hurting.* In so doing, we chip away at old patterns and, quite single-handedly, break them down. This will very likely surprise the other person (whether they show it or not) and it may just gear things in a different direction.

We disarm by dis-arming.

We still feel the way we feel about the issue. Our dueling partner still feels the way that they do. It just doesn't have to end up making everyone leave the exchange feeling worse off for having entered it.

In time, communication will inevitably improve. What is the harm, aside from a bit of effort, in making another feel more embraced? And how comforting if somebody of-fered this back to us?

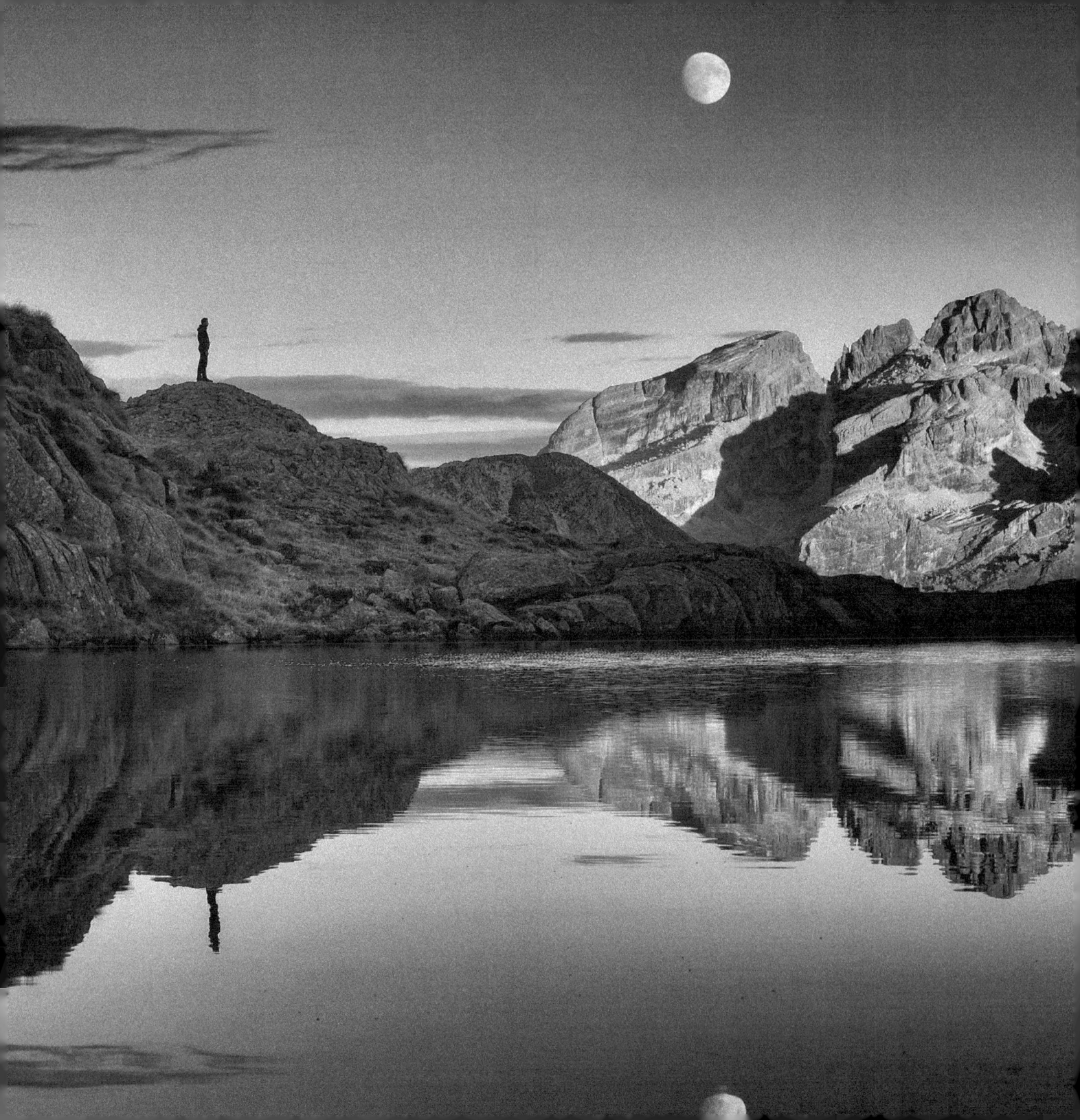

Noting Life

Meditation is not a blank mind.

The perception that it is is a total myth.

The continual stream of thought, emotion, and sensation from moment to moment is not an error. The notion that to find inner peace we must push away all mental workings and stare into some sort of nothingness *is* absolutely erroneous. We are hard wired (for survival's sake) to receive and process stimuli, and our lived environment is full of, is *entirely*, stimuli—whether gross or subtle, whether within or without.

Now that that's out of the way, let's talk about noting. Noting is one of the more foundational techniques of training the mind. If nothing else, it gives us something to do while meditating.

It's this simple: whenever we become distracted, or lost in thought, we make a (gentle) mental note of whatever it is that comes up, by categorizing it. A thought appears. Instead of following its story, we simply note it—"That's a thought"—and we let it go. A physical manifestation of emotion comes up and we begin to focus on it—notice it— "I'm holding my breath." Then call it what it is—"That's frustration, a feeling"—and we let it go. Remember, we need not note everything that comes into our minds, only those elements that really capture our attention and really pull us away from the object of focus.

Sometimes, the letting go can manifest as looking at the thing directly as it disappears on its own. Most often, we are reminded to come back to the breath. Notice it, softly name it as a matter of fact, and release it without any further thought. As though the thought/emotion/sensation were a bubble which lightly bursts the moment it is touched and noting is that featherlight touch. The breath is a useful anchor to consciously place the mind between this and that mental artifact. Back to the breath. Notice and let go. Back to the breath. Notice and let go. Like all things, practice really does make progress here.

In actual fact, this technique's greatest power may not be so much in supplying us with the *what to do*, but rather in preventing the *what not to do*. It directs the mind away from all the places it likes to lazily grasp: away from the rote, unhelpful, sometimes toxic automations that keep it weak and vulnerable to things outside of our control.

Here is the real secret: the thing that keeps us at arm's length from mental liberation (the thing that makes us think we just aren't good at meditating) is *identifying* with objects of attention.

Read that again.

It's *identification* with thoughts, sensations and/or emotions that is the pathology, not the thoughts, sensations and/or emotions themselves. This has taken me many years to understand. It's the latching onto these things— the mental fixations—that precludes our ability to see and think clearly and to feel calm, contented, and powerful.

While we may think that we are neither fixated nor unclear, every time we unconsciously follow a thought or hook into an emotion for seconds, for hours, for months at a time, we are both things. When we momentarily lose touch with what's right here right now, we strengthen dissociative brain pathways. When we don't remember how we got from point A to point B or haven't heard what was just said for being "in our heads," we have absolutely disconnected ourselves from the inherent newness (read, the hope and possible joy) of every passing moment that transpires therein.

Once again, as with most things in medicine, just because it's exceedingly common to identify with mental constructs in this way, it doesn't mean it's healthy.

To repeat this reframe: all of the constructs we may note within a formal or informal meditation practice are simply *objects of attention*. They are not something to judge or analyze nor are they instruments to gauge the success or failure of that particular practice. Importantly, they are neither "me" nor "not me." They just are.

Instead of trying to force our minds into blankness (reminder: not happening) or berating ourselves for following the thought, we can regularly practice techniques such as noting, in order to learn how *not* to identify with these cognitions. Plainly, to become well.

In the same way that it is normal for these constructs to

continually appear, so too, the hurdles of life are to be always, ongoingly, expected. This is not an aberration. It is the human experience.

What if we took each new obstacle, noted it, and let go of our grasping?

Of course, worldly situations do not disappear by virtue of our willing them so. While some aspects of experience may be in our control, many aren't. What is on the table here is our level of awareness of the various objects of attention and the nature of our approach. Can we sit through the experience, aware of the thoughts, emotions, and sensations that are arising as they are arising, and note them, too, as they are falling away? Is it possible to *not identify* with something that feels so personal, so unequivocally *ours?* Reframe. Remember. Everything is just occurring. And we are noting it.

If we practice doing this, in real time and on an ongoing basis, then it's entirely possible to feel less overwhelmed by the passing tide and infinitely more rooted. We may even find ourselves smiling confidently, mid-cyclone.

This level of resilience may seem far-fetched. Let me assure you, it is totally within reach. It's a choice. One we have to continue to make, again and again, toward conscious contentment.

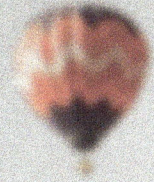

The thing that keeps us at arm's length from mental liberation… is identifying with objects of attention.

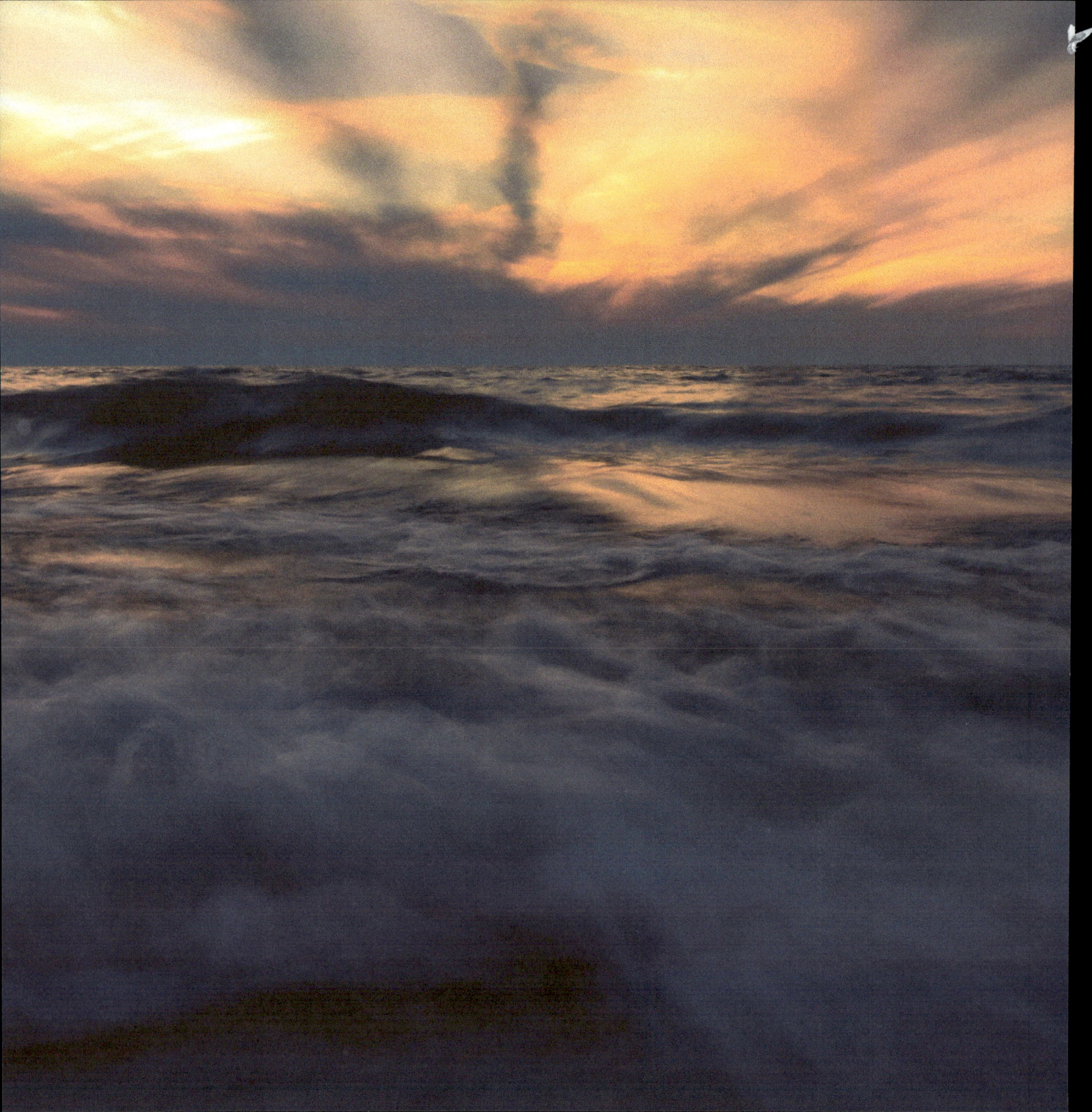

Navigating Change

The only thing constant is change.

This is a mantra I have been repeating to myself and to anyone who would listen, for a long time now. I believe it was written by a Greek philosopher named Heraclitus. He is said to have written it in a book that was destroyed and found only in fragments.

I believe what our Grecian thinker was saying was that we can hold as certain that whatever life circumstance we find ourselves in, whatever weather, it will inevitably be different fifteen minutes from now, an hour from now, a week from now.

Still, knowing that change is coming doesn't mean that we know when it's coming or what form it will take. The complete ambiguity surrounding all facets of that change—its onset, presentation, character, shape, amplitude—is a blessing in disguise. As much as we think we'd love to know what's coming and when (so that we can plan for it, good or bad), we never can, and that's actually helpful. It's this unpredictability which forces us to stay present with what is happening here and now, whether we are loving these feelings or circumstances or not.

While, in hard times, this adage might feel like a light-house in a storm, it's also possible that the same truth can provoke fear and anxiety if we happen to be in the midst of happier times.

The problem is in how we define and thus understand the language used. If we perceive change in binary terms, then only opposing extremes exist. If things are good now, just wait, they will inevitably turn sour. When it feels life has thrown us under the bus, the issues are bound to fully resolve.

If we just take off these 0 and 1 glasses and understand that everything in between also classifies as change, ah, well now we've got a much greater appreciation for the vast opportunity that is held within this mantra.

Are we in a satisfying, loving relationship we hope will never end? Are we out of work, mid-divorce, unfulfilled, unwell, generally in dire straits? All these things will undergo *modification*. Some in small, gradual, interesting ways we could never have anticipated. Some suddenly, and with great drama. Some external circumstances will shift as we grow and what we may have thought we wanted, too, changes alongside these.

The fact is, we don't know how our situation will change, in what way, to what extent, or when. There is tremendous solace to be found in this. Despite our best efforts at projection, we just cannot know. All we can do is understand that we don't understand, stop prognosticating, and work on this, here, today. Notice and play an active role.

Through those rough moments, expect that that isn't *it*.

There is a great emotional burden that we tack onto already-difficult moments when we repeatedly ask ourselves: "Is this how it's going to be forever? Is this how I'm going to feel? Will this loneliness persist? This anger? This resent, guilt, depression, anxiety… is this how it will always be?" And like any line of thinking, we strengthen it the more we identify with it. They are questions, sure, but leading ones. And though we may never frankly answer them, when our brain is involved in asking this again and again, it fills in the answer it's being led toward—yes. *Yes*, it believes, *this is likely how it will always be*. The more these ideas cross our minds, the more we believe them to be true statements.

Unfortunately, that false answer is the difference between having the strength to overcome something and full-on, hopeless resignation. We really are equipped to tolerate so much… so long as we can know for certain that an end—read, a change—is around the proverbial corner.

Where we can get ourselves to accept that change always inevitably comes, that's the birthplace of resilience and hope and making it through, all the stronger.

If we think back to a time of emotional rock-bottomedness, when our expectations or dreams were in severe opposition to our lived reality, that was the moment we broke. Or rather, that we *felt broken*. Had we understood then that the very nature of our ocean *is* waves crashing, tides rising and receding, calm waters, and everything in between, how much more yielding and receptive could we have been?

All we can do is understand that we don't understand, stop prognosticating, and work on this, here, today.

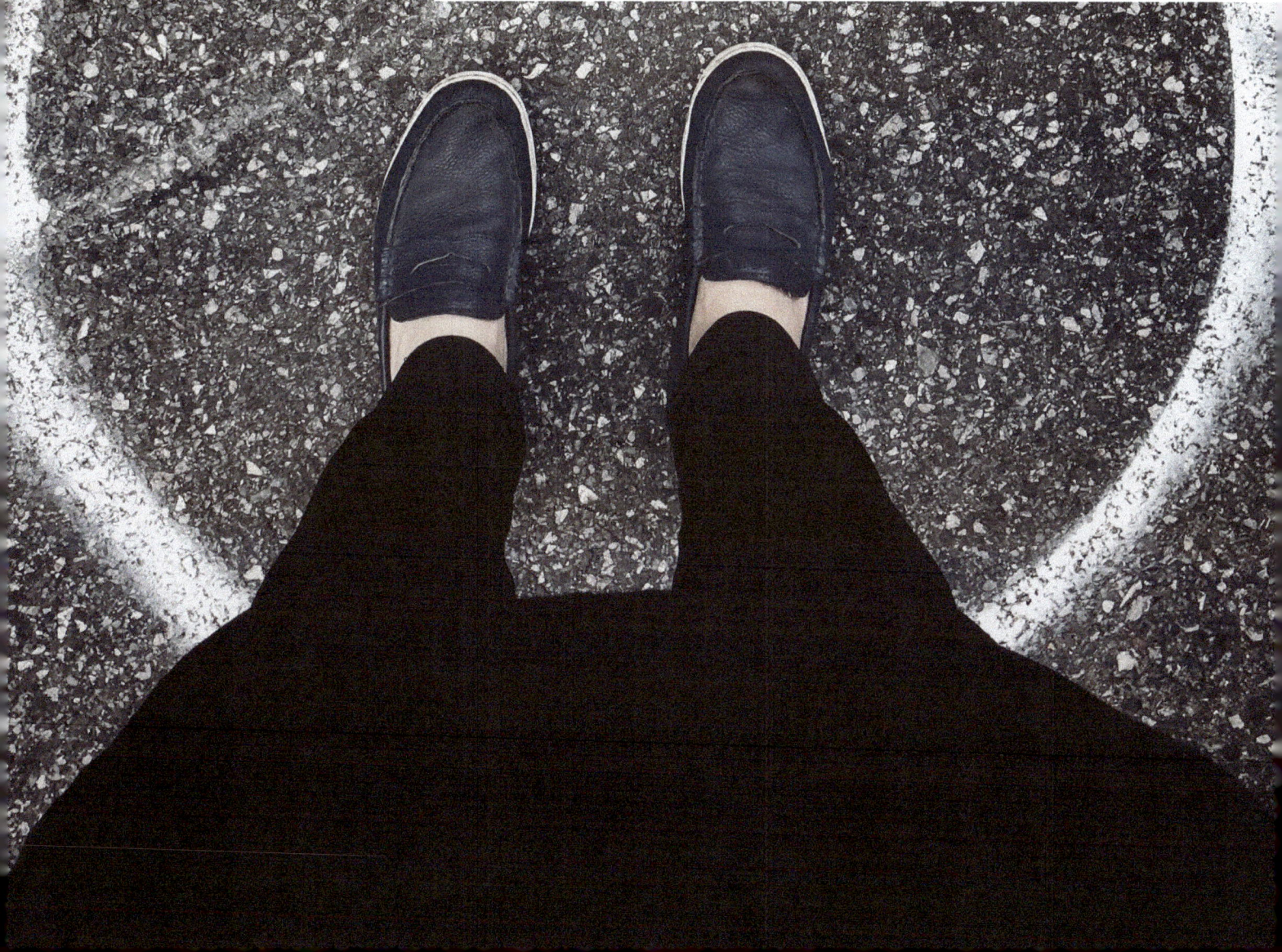

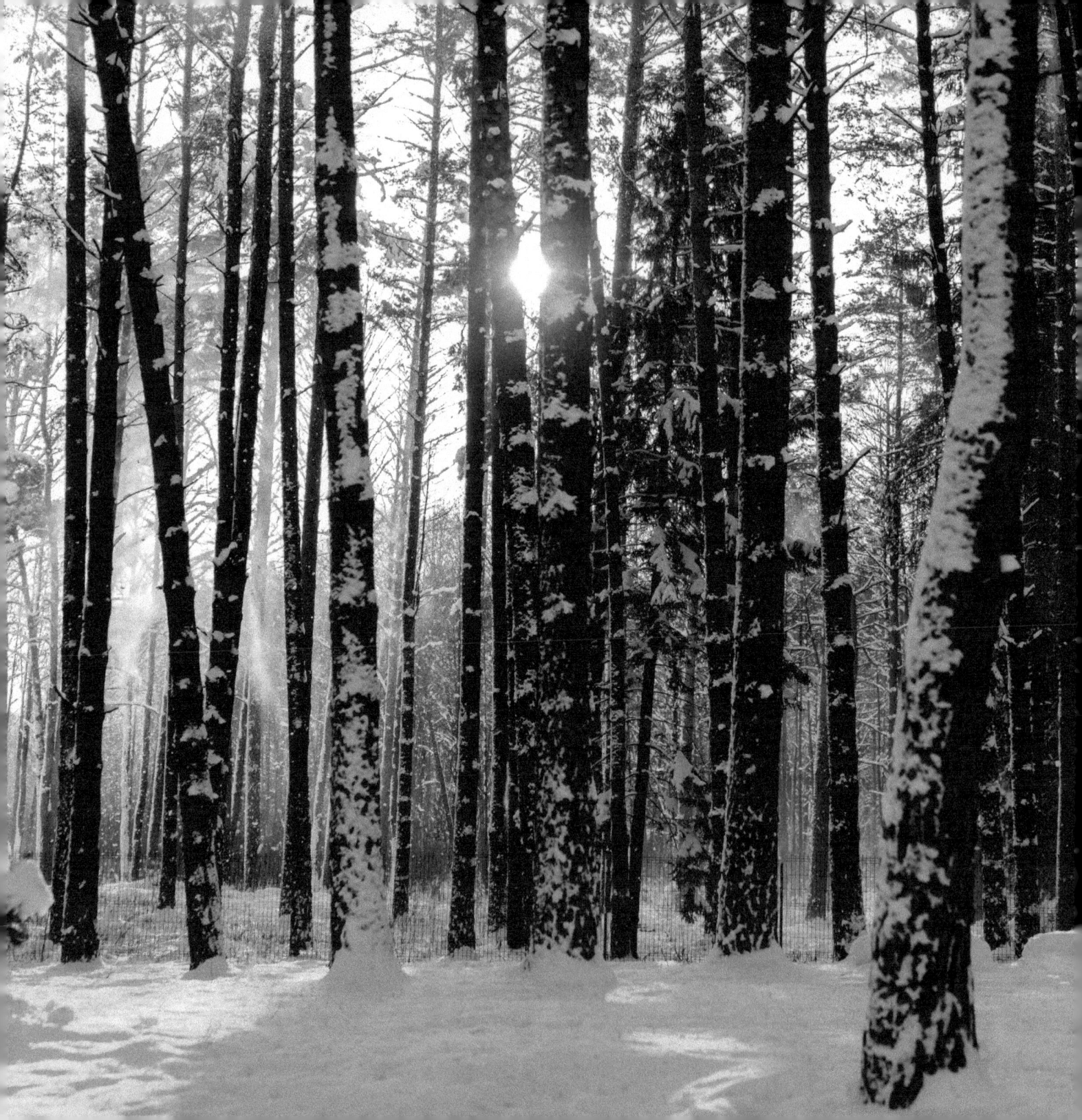

Practicing Integrity

There is a clear parallel that can be drawn between the anatomical integrity required of a yoga pose and the cognitive-emotional-behavioural integrity we must demand within ourselves to live a fulfilling life.

When you're a beginner in yoga, everybody tells you, "Just keep at it. Be where your body's at and things will evolve. You will see a progression." This is very true. You keep at it. You keep coming back to the mat. You keep returning to the same poses, and you will inevitably see progress. But this inevitability comes with an asterisk. The asterisk denotes that this evolution comes only when practicing with integrity.

In the context of a yoga pose, integrity looks like alignment. The spine is a great starting point in assessing whether or not we're in alignment. And to be clear, alignment where the spine is concerned is not a straight line of vertebrae stacked perfectly on top of one another. We have natural curvatures, slightly different from one person to the next, which when perfectly aligned have the fewest overall tensions pulling it in one direction or another. A foundational posture to get a sense of our spine is neutral standing, or, Mountain pose [see "Tadasana" in the Yoga section]. Are we over-curving or under-curving anywhere? Are we jutting out our neck? Compressing in the low back? Your standing pose will necessarily look a bit different to the person next to you in class—our bones, joints, muscles, and angles between are our own and are rarely, if ever, "textbook."

A close second to the spinal column as an alignment tool is the stacking of other joints. Generally, in any pose, feeling for how large and small joints are positioned on top of one another is a helpful way to begin to train our proprioceptive sense. Proprioception is an awareness of our body in space; for example, the ability to know exactly where your foot is without looking at it. Stacking shoulder over elbow over wrist, for example. Or hip over knee over ankle. At times, a pose requires a closed hip (keeping it at the level of the sacrum, which usually means dropping the raised hip somewhat); in other poses, we open it up to stack the two hip joints vertically. Focusing on this kind of anatomical alignment—rather than how 'advanced' our pose looks in the studio mirror—is how we safely move our bodies and find that inevitable development that comes with a dedicated yoga practice.

The thinking that the pose must look a certain way (that our leg need lift *this high*) to be doing yoga, is a notion we must throw out the window at the outset. When a teacher asks you to "listen to your body" and "be where you're at," there is an actual, useful instruction beneath those platitudes, trust me. When we pull back or lean in more deeply in response to the messages our body is sending us, we not only prevent injury but progress further, and faster.

So, maybe I succeed at raising my leg all the way up there and there is acute pain, or I have to hold my breath to achieve it, or the only way up is to lose my spinal alignment.

221

Here, getting the pose to look a certain way, zeroing in on one flashy element and forgetting the foundational rest, has broken all of its honesty. It's a shape, but it ceases to be a posture.

For our practice to be honest, we need to show up knowing that it changes day to day and hour to hour. One might ask, *Can I breathe in this position?* We will be breathing with effort, surely, but where can we breathe and stay for a while? Is it possible to hold this pose for ten slow breaths or longer? We could make this a sort of litmus test for postural integrity.

If we are truly "listening to our bodies" in the present moment, the look of the pose will always be different, however gross or fine these changes. I'll posit that it is of far greater value to *feel* the rightness of the posture rather than to see it.

This physical aspect of alignment is crucial. It isn't, however, the only one.

If lining up one's joints, spine and breath meets the behavioral requirements, how do we integrate the mental (thoughts) and emotional (feelings) facets of true alignment, on and off the mat? Inside a yoga class, this equates to checking in with how we are feeling on that day, within each pose as well as within each mindful transition.

How much or how little sleep did we get the night prior? How affected are we currently by the tensions at home or work? To what extent have we been holding self-care as sacred or as dispensable? It's about asking ourselves what we really need in that moment and always riding the fine line between a healthy push and a gentle pull. Sometimes it truly is Child's Pose we need to lie in (nurturing grounding, cooling, and yin) regardless of what the rest of the class is doing. Sometimes what we need is to get past our mental blocks and actually attempt to stay in that nemesis Chaturanga or Dancer's Pose (nurturing energy, heat and yang).

Off the mat, when living our non-yoga lives (as if there were such a thing!), we can foster true integrity when our actions align with our words, with how we are feeling in that moment, as well as with the values and beliefs we hold close.

Ever tell a little white lie, no malice intended, to save time, save face, or for no reason? It's not a huge lie.

Sometimes we get away with these. They end as quickly as they began. Other times, they collect. Something happens, someone questions, and we feel we have to repeat the lie or tell a different one to keep the story consistent.

There may be a tiny nudge of off-feeling, but it's tolerable. On rare occasions, it snowballs in a harmful direction.

As soon as we are a little bit out of alignment—when our behaviors and words are out of tune with one another and/or with what we believe—we've lost integrity. Now, something is apt to breakdown. We threaten or lose a close relationship. We feel irritable and don't know why.

We pull a hamstring, we get caught in a lie.

Like everything else, this integrity thing is a practice. Are we walking our talk? Talking our walk? The first item of business is learning to read the cues our physical, mental, and emotional bodies are speaking. It's the difference between stretching and straining. The difference between the knot in your stomach that comes from without and the one that comes from within. The only way to become intimately connected to our own wondrous language (in all its dialects) is to pay attention.

Stacked vertebrae. Pelvis and chin tucked slightly under in keeping the natural curvatures of the spine. Alignment, Integrity.

We get a little taller, we move with more ease.

Feeling stronger, more confident.

Feeling well.

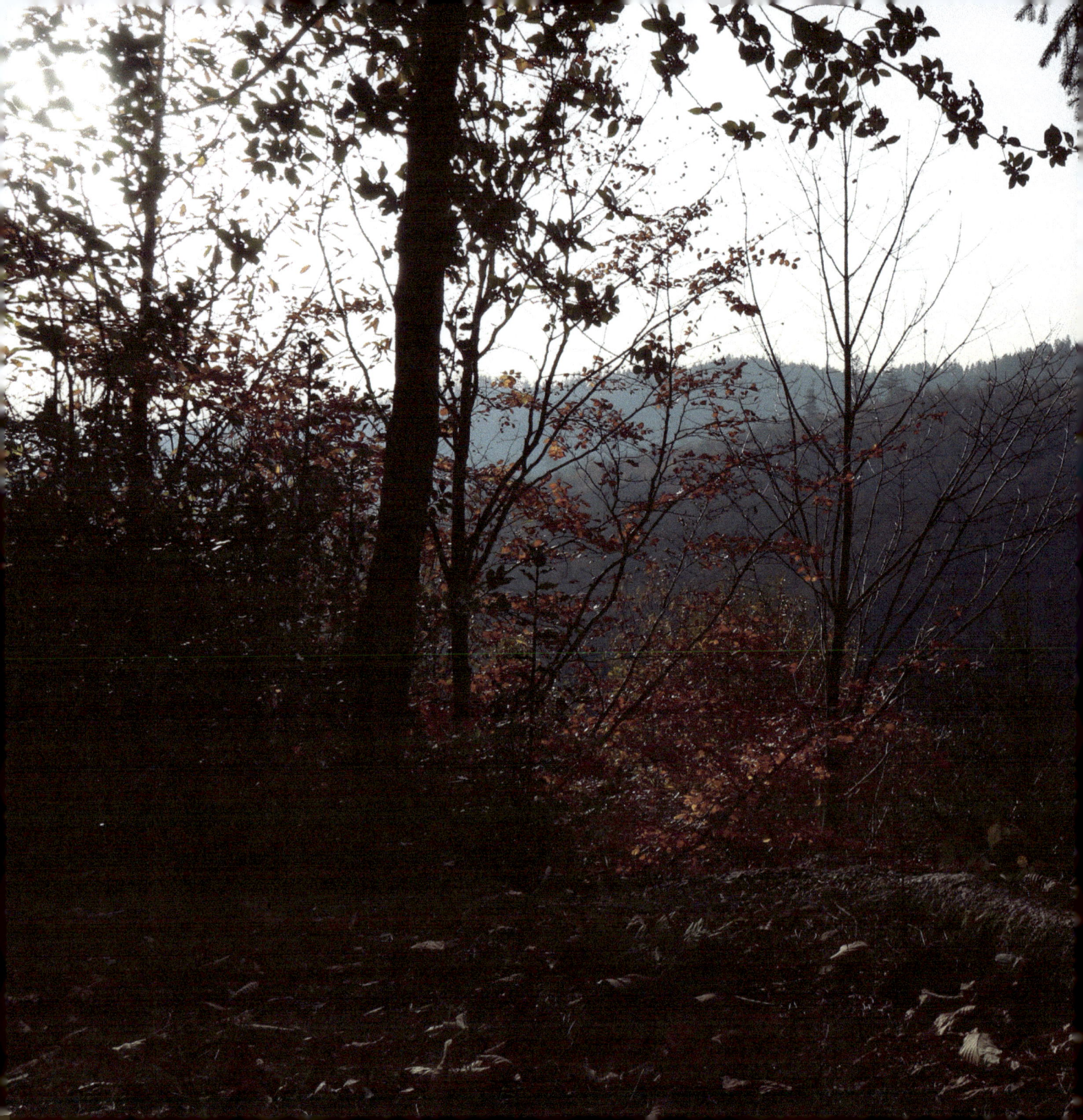

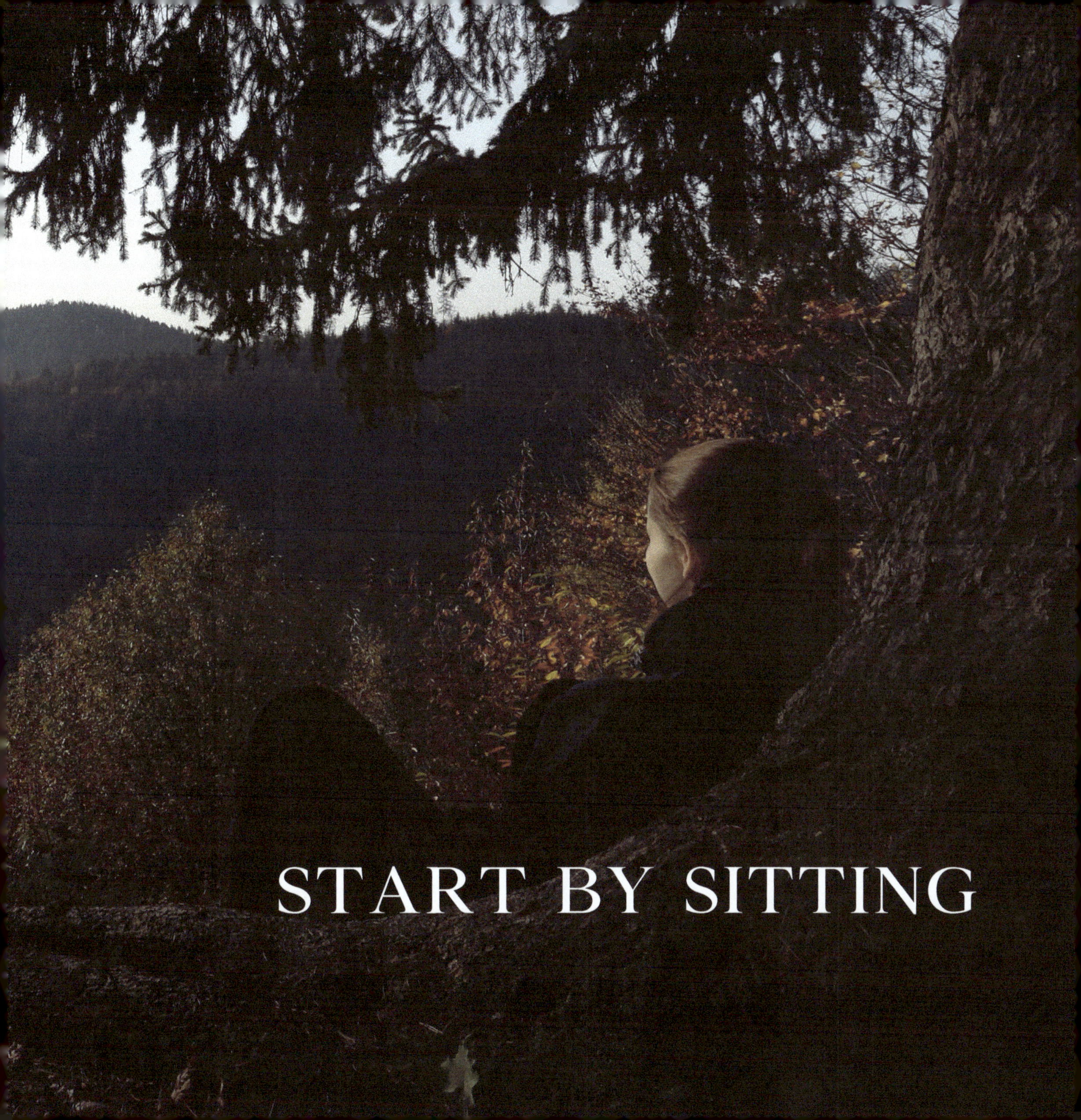

START BY SITTING

So HOW do I even start meditating?

I don't have the time, I have no idea what I'm doing, what's the point anyway?

Any of this sound familiar?

Start by sitting.

The answers will all come in time. For now, just trust that so much research supports it and people the world over are finding massive benefit. No need to query things further than open yourself and see.

But how?

There are many amazing apps, books, programs, and resources out there to help guide you. For now, start with this. Commit to seven days of sitting with attention. There is nothing that you can do that is right or wrong. The only thing is to try to bring awareness to the minutes of your practice. I'll guide you.

Take a comfortable seat. I suggest sitting, not lying down, as lying down tends to invite us into slumber (go figure?). Sleep, while a wonderful, health-promoting practice, is unfortunately not a meditation. For attention, we want to cultivate a gentle, calm awareness.

And to be aware, we must be awake. Sit down on a chair, on the floor on a block or a pillow; whatever puts your body at most ease to minimize distractions. Just see where your mind goes.

Set a timer for five minutes. Find somewhere quiet. Though finding a quiet space is certainly not a requisite for meditation, in the early stages, you may find it helpful. Observe. Start there. Begin to notice certain thoughts or emotions arising as well as physical sensations. If you're feeling particularly scattered and/or your mind is racing, you may find it beneficial to choose one thing to become attentive to, to focus the mind. The feeling of your hands in your lap or of your back against the chair. The way your chest rises and falls in respiration or the sensation of breath under the nose are good options. Another technique that can anchor your mind at the outset of practice or anytime in the middle is to silently count the breaths (up to ten and back down again for one round). See if you can tune in, heighten your senses.

This is simply a commitment to putting the time aside, to getting a bit quiet and to noticing. That's all.

Commit to a short goal—to seven days. Maybe this is all completely new to you. If so, a heartfelt welcome. Possibly you are an experienced meditator but need something to bring you back to dedicated practice and remind you of why you sit.

The best time to start is right now. Trust me that when you plan less and, instead, jump in, you're ninety percent there. It's like tying your shoes and being out the door before a walk or run. It's in the bag. If you wait until just the right time to begin, full of excuses as to why this moment isn't quite right for you, believe me, you have never needed it more than this moment.

And just one gut-check before proceeding: If you've ever told yourself or others that you just don't have the time, that you truly cannot set aside five to ten minutes daily—"at least not right now"—make a tally of where you are spending your waking minutes. Are they all indispensable, every last one? Surely, you aren't scrolling social nor watching TV for ten minutes or more daily. Surely, not that.

I'll repeat: *The best time to start is right now.*

[For each of the following seven days, read the corresponding prompt for that day, prior to starting your timer. Read it twice if you'd like, but don't skip ahead, only one day's prompt at a time. Then put the book down, hit 'start' and close your eyes to begin]

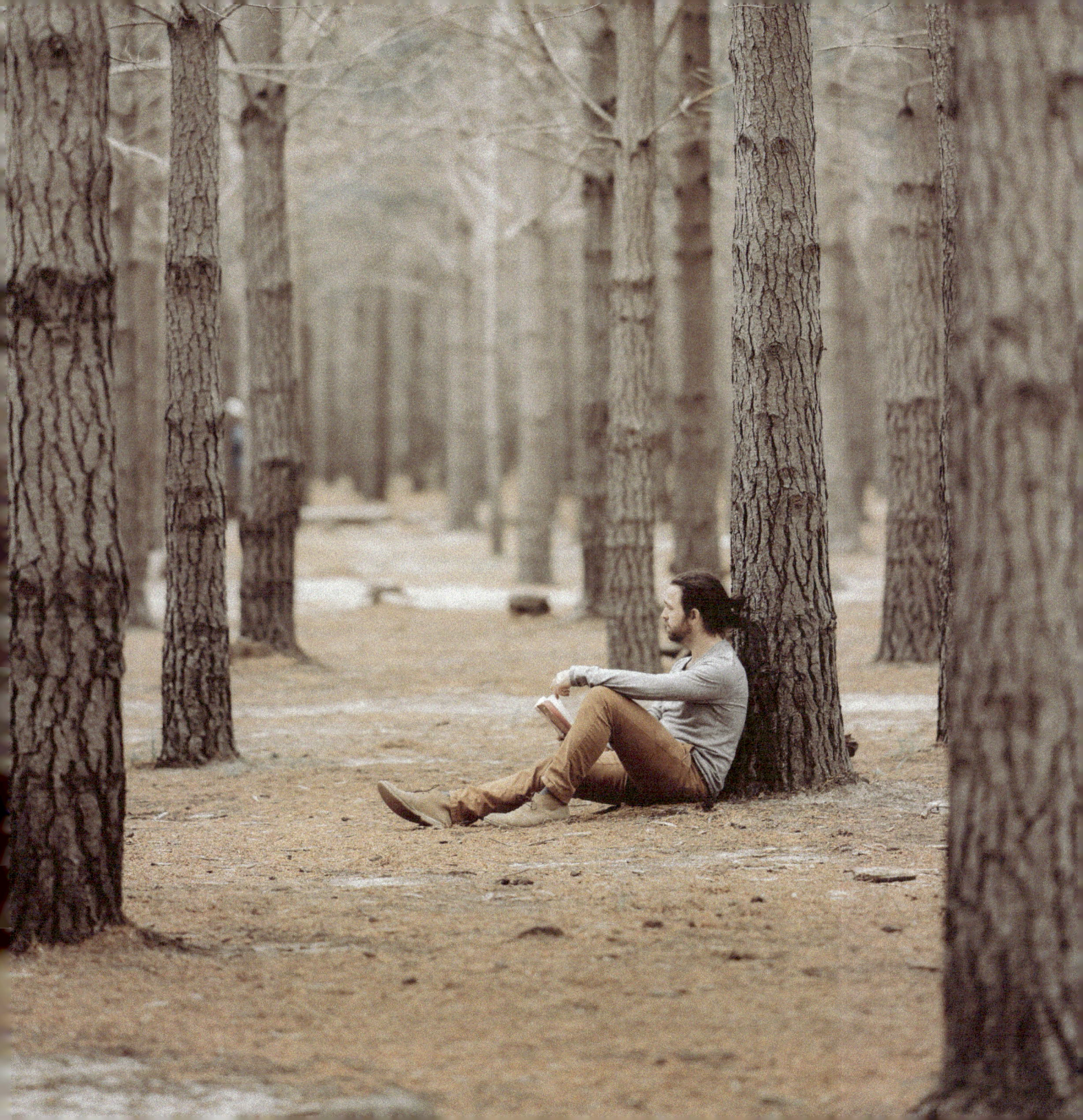

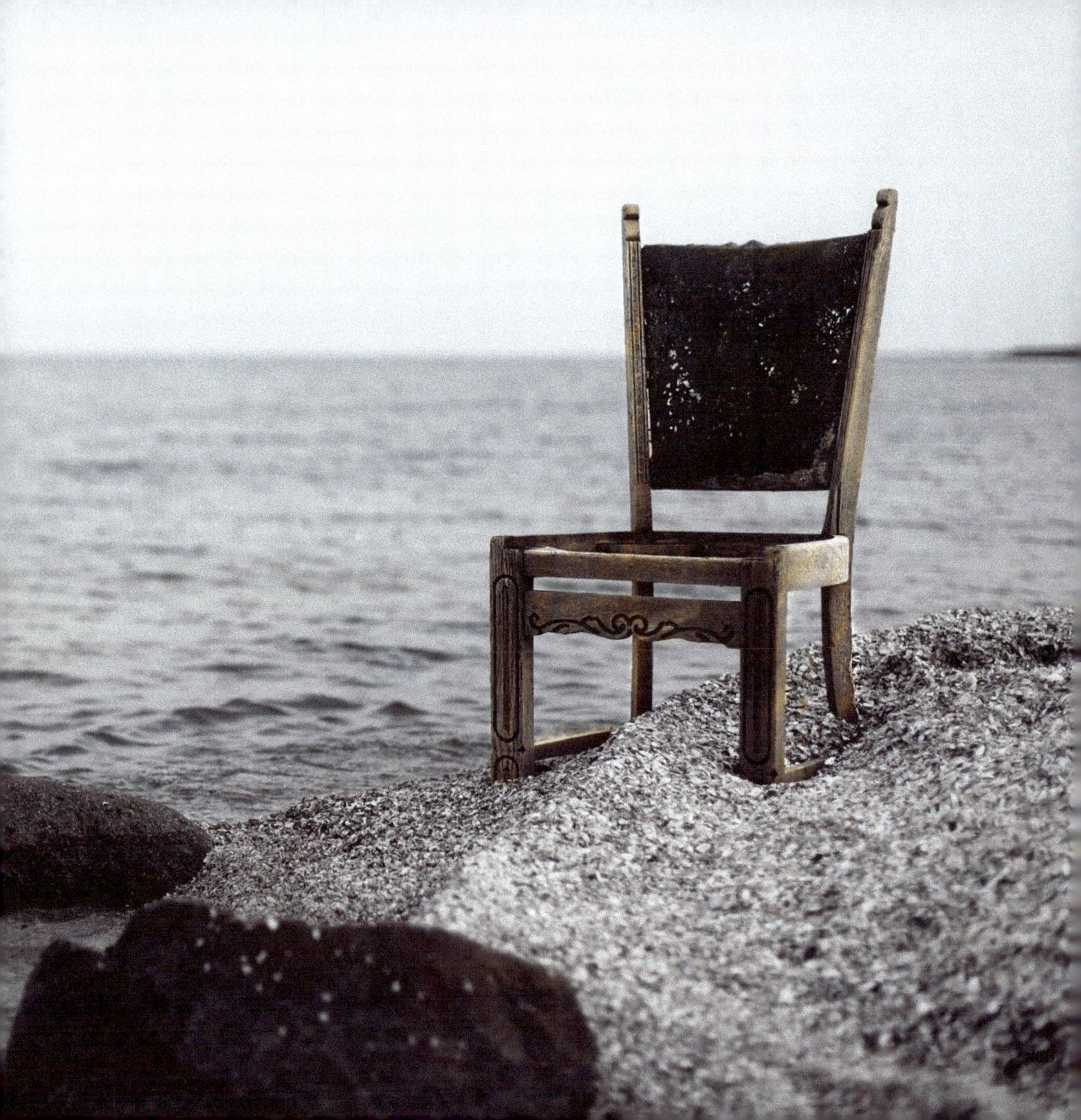

Day One

It begins here.

Sit for five minutes, at some point today.

Find a comfortable chair and sit with both feet planted, back straight.

If the floor is your thing, sit however makes your back and body comfortable. Having a cushion or block beneath your sitting bones to lift the back of your seat is often very helpful.

Sit. And just notice what you notice. See if you can notice without judgment.

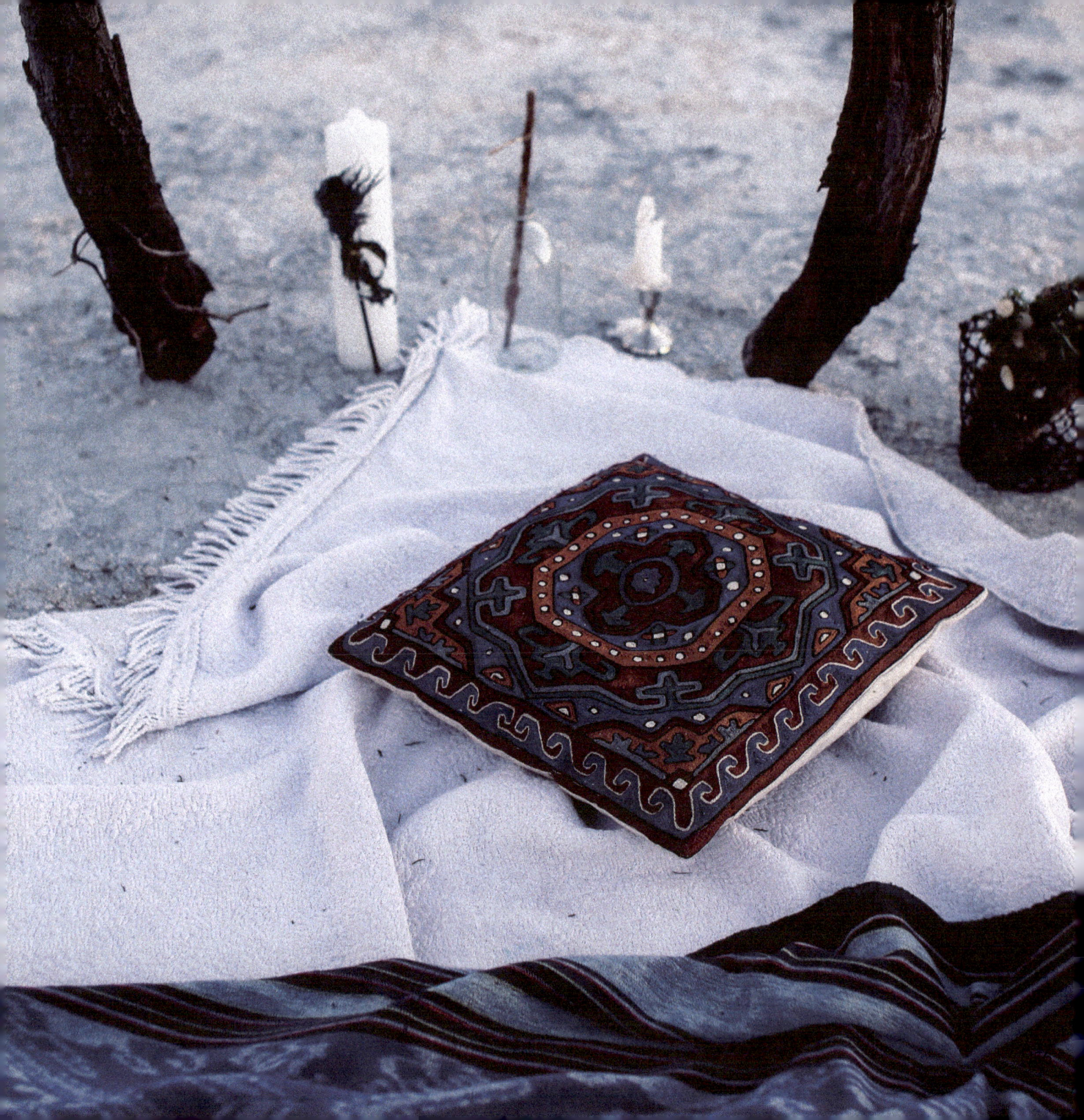

Day Two

Show up again.

How did yesterday go?

Did it feel too long? Did it go by like a blur, while distracted in to-do lists or events of that week? Was it peaceful or blah or uncomfortably close to yourself?

Try to take the first few moments of sitting to pay attention to the world around you—sounds, temperature, movements—and then decide to turn that inward.

Anything and everything is ok and exactly right, for you, right now.

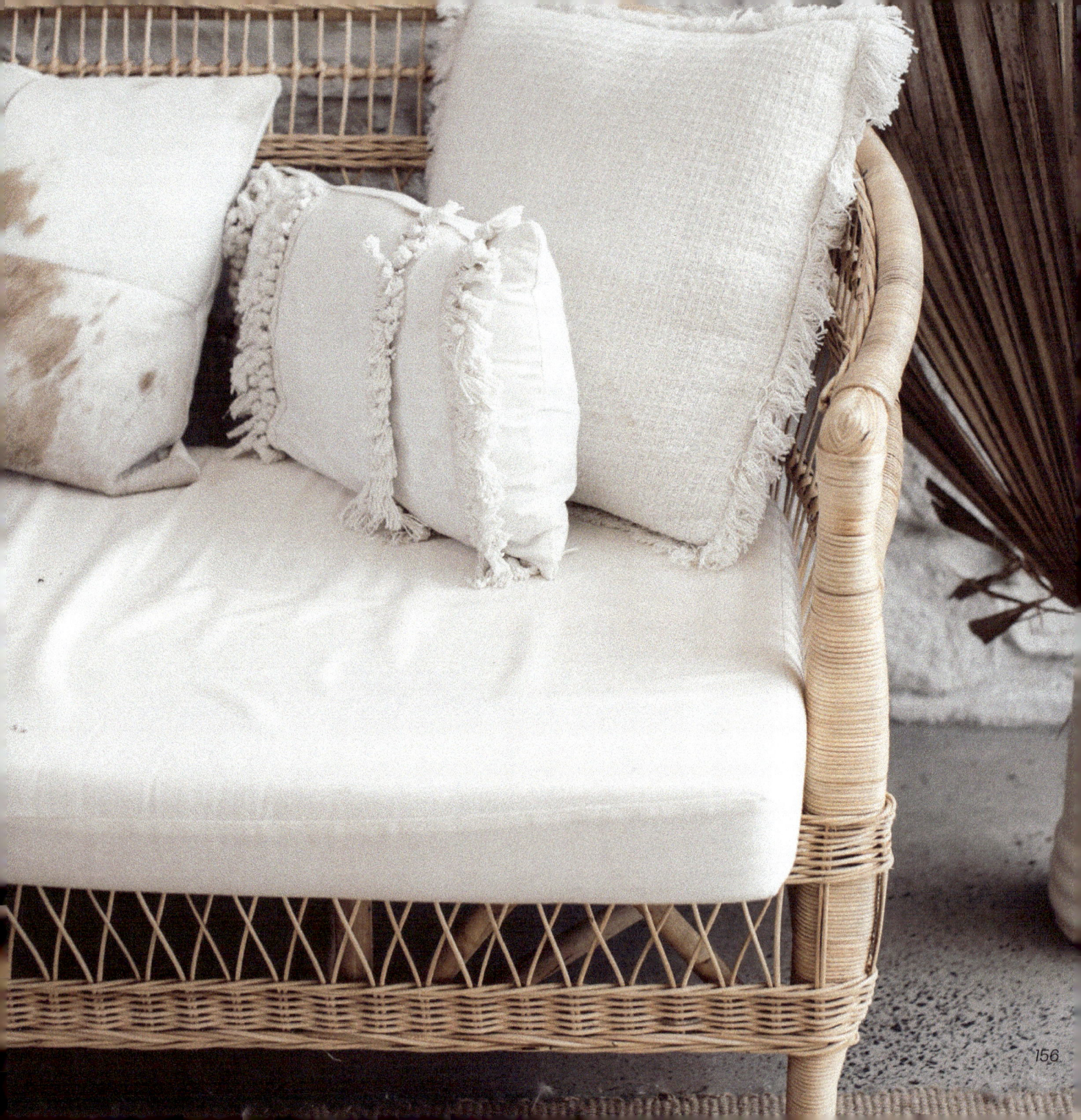

Day Three

If you missed yesterday, it's ok.

Come on back.

How did it feel, transitioning from external attention to internal? Helpful / not helpful, easy, challenging?

Try noticing each exhale, from its beginning to its end. See if that keeps you present. Once again, no need to try to change the breathing pattern, but rather, notice it. Pay attention to the evolution of your breath within the span of the next five to ten minutes. You may find it has distinctly changed at the end of the session without even trying. If not, you're ok. You didn't do it wrong. Note it. Move on.

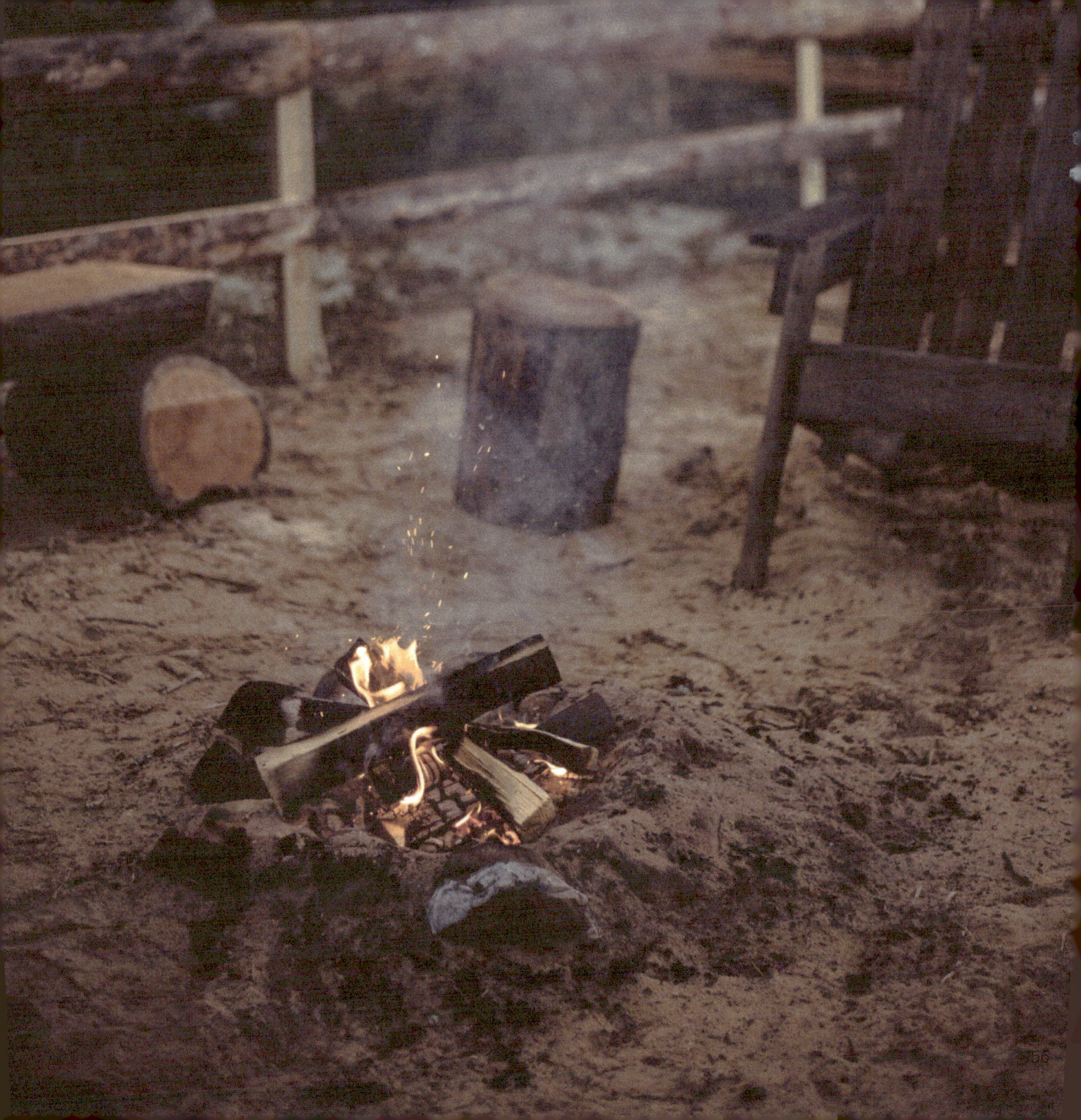

Day Four

Over halfway, friends.

As with other goals, you may have started off strong and committed... possibly still there, but just as possibly feeling any or all the following:

- This is a waste of my time, nothing is happening
- I already missed a day or two, I might as well
  forget it altogether
- My mind is all over the place, I'm not doing it right
- I can't concentrate, even for five minutes
- I'm sure this works for other people, but for me it
  only makes things worse
- I'm stressed enough as it is

... Anyone?

Come back to your seat. Trust the process. If you want anything to change in your life, you will have to start by doing something different. In this case, sticking to this goal, even if you don't understand where it could possibly go.

There is no room for scrutiny or appraisal. No room for judgment within you nor upon this community of readers. Cheer one another on, as I am doing with all my heart— most of all, cheer *yourself* on.

Now come on back and SIT.

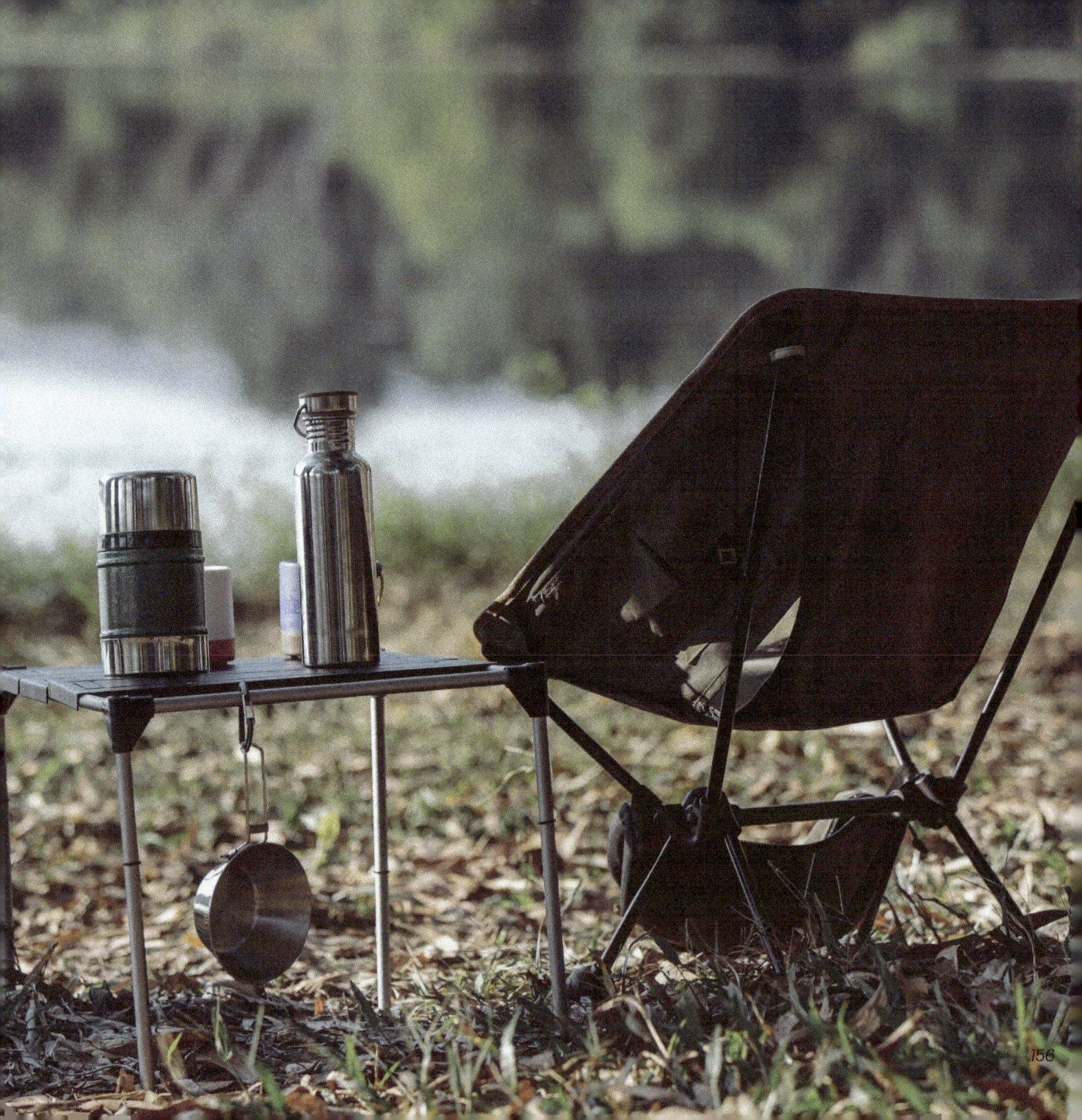

Day Five

Take your seat.

It's a brand-new day. Let go of anything that did or did not happen for you in the days since this challenge began.

Consider the phrase, "It didn't sit right". Give this a second. We take an idea or explanation and check it—as though testing an unknown key into our own personal lock.

What does it mean if something, conversely, *does* "sit right"?

In our comfortable seat, when we've accounted for our body, our time, our space, our needs... When we are quiet of mind and free from distraction, we are *sitting right*.

There, we are in alignment—in our intuition, our truest self, our home within.

Today, gently notice whatever comes up as it appears and then disappears.

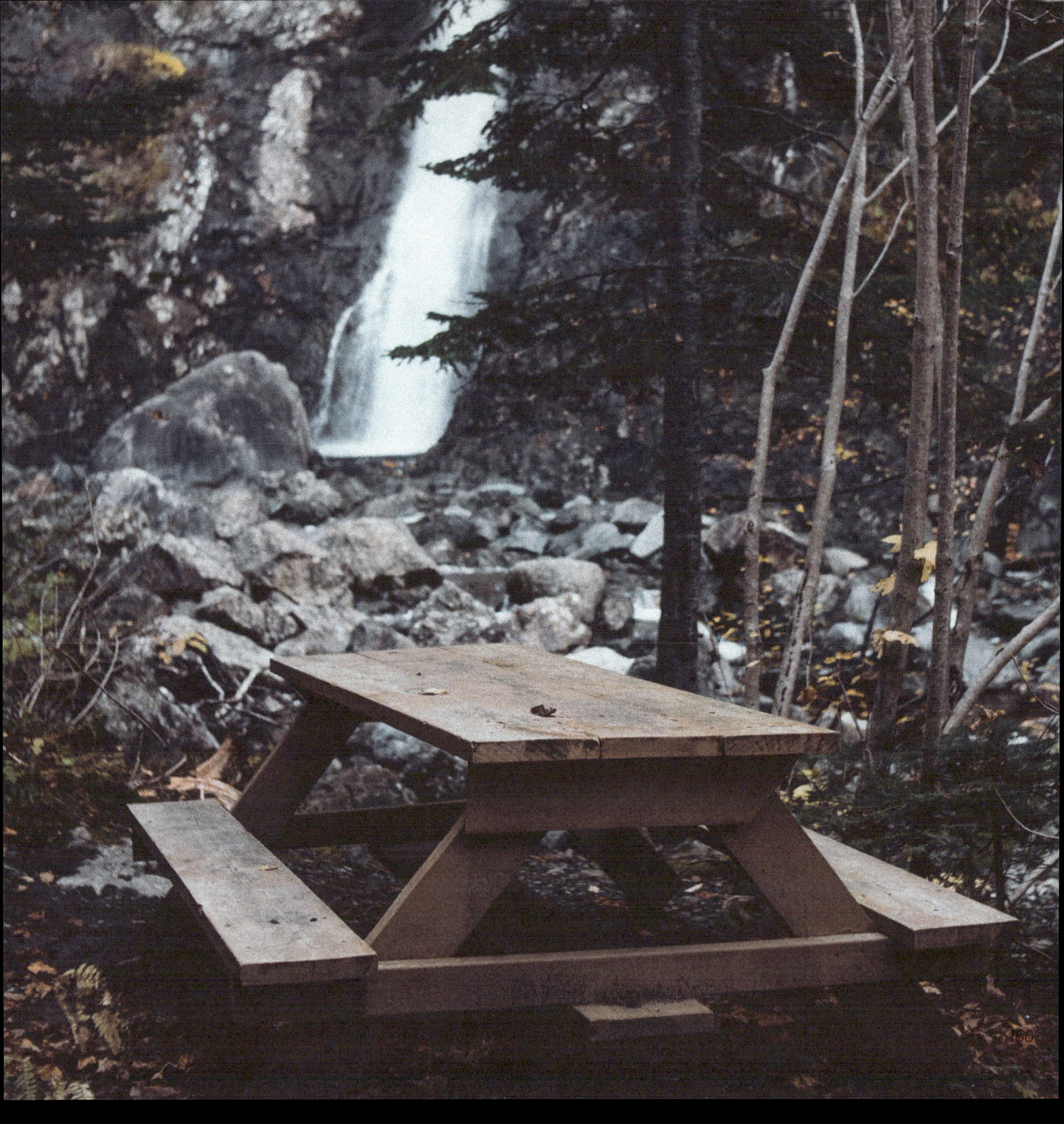

Day Six

Are you still with me?

If the attention practice is beginning to feel boringly rote, there are two things you could consider:

1 - Continued, consistent repetition is a simple yet powerful way to learn a new skill,

and

2 - The concept of Beginner's Mind will be your greatest defense against boredom, ever. It's an attitude of mind. Simply, it means that no matter where you are in your evolution of practice, you come back every day to sit as though for the first time:

- with no expectations as to how this is going to go / how you will feel, etc. (without prior experience, the canvas is blank; the possibilities are truly endless)

- with no prior knowledge about anything (even if you are a well-practiced monk!), imagine what you could learn?

Approach your daily practice with these things in mind. Each return is a new day of your course. We can have no idea what each class will bring.

Now, sit quietly again, as though opening a door to a completely new experience. No biases, no expectations.

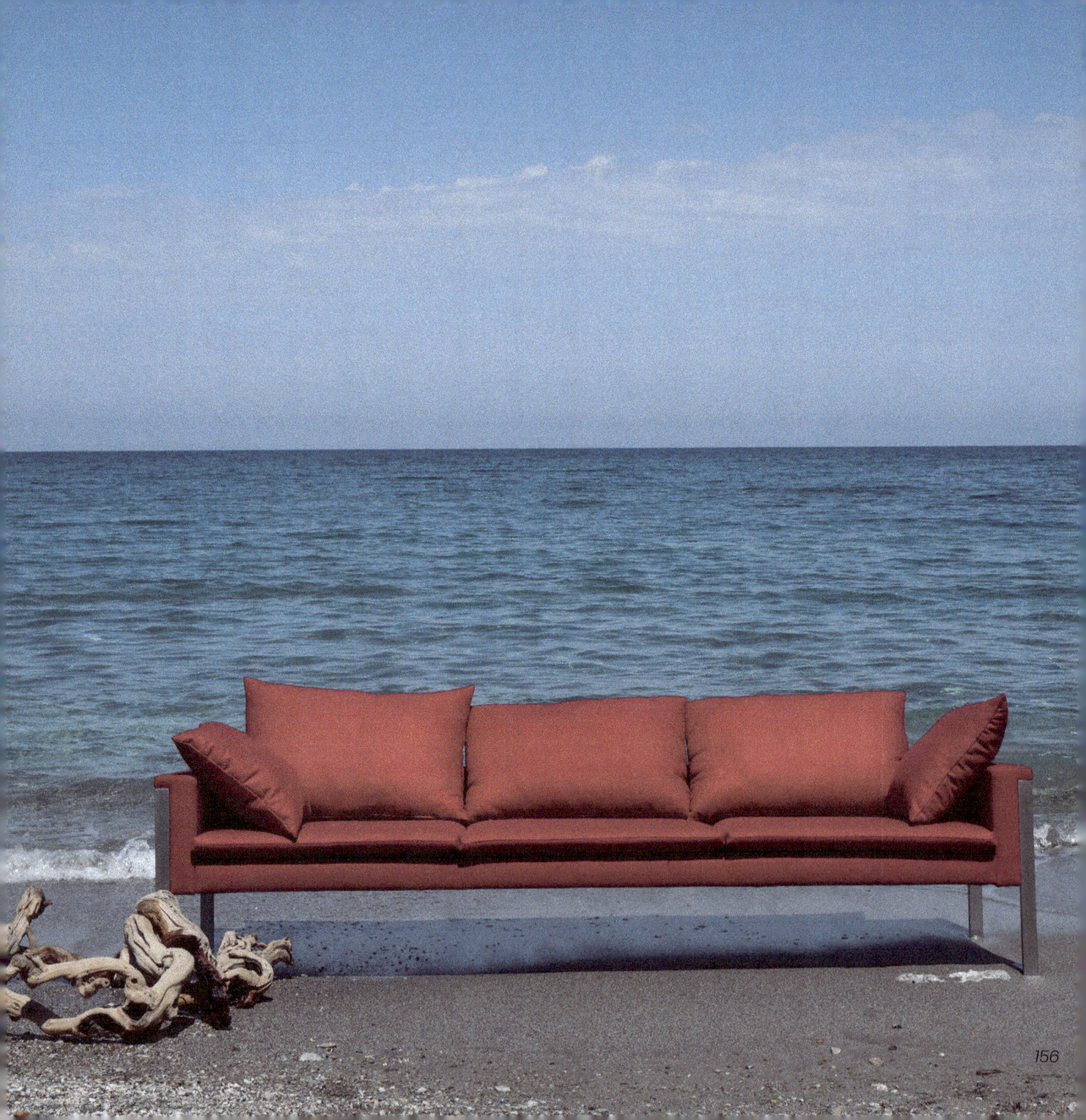

Day Seven

Final day of the challenge, and just the beginning.

If you've stuck with this (whether you missed a couple of days or not), I am so incredibly proud of you for showing up. Let this short but powerful commitment you just made be not only the beginning of an attention/mindfulness/meditation practice, let it be the beginning of prioritizing the commitments you make to yourself.

This is the very best gift you could ever give to yourself, your partner, your children, your family, and friends: that of prioritizing *you*. Asserting your worth, and at the same time modeling this for others.

After you've completed your five or ten minutes today, take a moment to pause and reflect before moving on with the rest of your day. Commit to seeing this training course through. Daily doses, however short, need to be to be consistent to become part of your psyche in any measurable way. You miss a day, or two, no matter. Heck, you missed a few years? Let it go, unequivocally and absolutely. Decide to fully relieve yourself of any analysis or evaluation. Just come back. Recommit every single time.

Seven days to get your feet wet, to carve out space in your day and see how scheduling in a break for self-care and self-work can feel. You may have already found something positive come out of this week, you may not have.

Like any course of study, we reap what we sow. And just like planting seeds, the efforts required here are not heroic. Some consistent water and sun, a little daily attention. There are profound learnings taking root. It's no exaggeration to note that, when nurtured, these have the power to positively shift every aspect of your life, in a relatively short amount of time.

The challenge may be over, but the joy has just begun.

Love and light my friends xx

Ana

"Everything that has a beginning, has an ending. Make your peace with that and all will be well."

Jack Kornfield

Photo Credits

FRONT COVER – S Migaj (Pexels)

CONTENTS – Dziana Hasanbekava (Pexels)

LANGUAGE

LANGUAGE (SECTION COVER) – Lachlan Ross (Pexels)
DRISHTI – Oleg Magni (Pexels)
EQUANIMITY – Josh Willink (Pexels)
PRANA – Ben Mack (Pexels)
MINDFULNESS – Marlon Martinez (Pexels)
MANTRA – Olga Lioncat (Pexels)
RUMINATION – Noah Silliman (StockSnap)
AHIMSA – Ugur Tandogan (Pexels)
NAMASTE – Eternal Happiness (Pexels)
VIPASSANA – Noelle Otto (Pexels)
EGO – Amine M'siouri (Pexels)

BUILDING AWARENESS

BUILDING AWARENESS (SECTION COVER) – Sam Kolder (Pexels)
BREATH – Anastasia Shuraeva (Pexels)
WORDS – Alina Vilchenko (Pexels)
MOOD – Trace Hudson (Pexels)
TENSION – Никита Семехин (Pexels)
EXPRESSION – Aadii (Pexels)
THOUGHTS – Laker (Pexels)
PREJUDICE – Anna Nekrashevich (Pexels)
SLEEP – Nine Koepfer (Unsplash)
BALANCE – Alexander Grigorian (Pexels)
PACE – Shahbaz Sheikh (Life of Pix)
GRATITUDE – Alexey Demidov (Pexels)
TRIGGERS – Rahul Pandit (Pexels)
IMPATIENCE – Henry & Co (Pexels)
STRENGTHS – Dmitriy Ganan (Pexels)

MASTER TEACHERS

MASTER TEACHERS (SECTION COVER) – Jens Johnsson (Pexels)
"The quieter you become..." (Anonymous) – Rachel Claire (Pexels)
"Do your practice and..." (K Pattabhi Jois) – Tima Miroshnichenko (Pexels)
"Fighting to preserve our mind..." (Venerable Chwasan) – Vlada Karpovich (Pexels)
"In the untrained mind..." (Jack Kornfield) – Torbjorn Sandbakk (Unsplash)
"We have never stayed home..." (Erich Schiffman) – Nachelle Nocom (Unsplash)
"The next message..." (Ram Das) – Hugh Han (Unsplash)
"Everything happens for you..." (Byron Katie) – Jacob Kelvinj (Pexels)
"The only way to live..." (Tara Brach) – Gianluca Grisenti (Pexels)
"Our actions almost always..." (Michael Stone) – Jeremy Bishop (Pexels)
"Your life doesn't get any better..." (Sam Harris) – Anete Lusina (Pexels)
"You are the sky..." (Pema Chodron) – Szabó Viktor (Pexels)
"Rather than being your thoughts..." (Eckhart Tolle) – Jeffrey Czum (Pexels)
"I believe that attention is..."(Gary Vaynerchuk) – Mathias P.R. Reding (Pexels)
"It is the power to focus..." (Patañjali) – Hedi Alija (Unsplash)
"The real meditation is..." (Jon Kabat-Zinn) – Eberhard Grossgasteiger (Pexels)
"Yoga does not remove us..." (Donna Farhi) – Ketut Subiyanto (Pexels)
"Move a muscle..." (Anonymous) – Inside Creative House (Shutterstock)
"Yoga has never been about..." (Seane Corn) – Body Bend Yoga (Nappy)
"Sometimes you need to sit..." (Charlotte Eriksson) – Kira Schwarz (Pexels)
"If we feed ourselves noise..." (Max Strom) – José Martín Ramírez Carrasco (Unsplash)
"Endure both..." (Geshe Chekawa) – Jarod Lovekamp (Pexels)
"Accept - then act..." (Eckhart Tolle) – Redd (Unsplash)
"An intellectual mind that is..." (BKS Iyengar) – Benin Lorenzo (Pexels)
"Love is the bridge..." (Rumi) – Kaique Rocha (Pexels)
"You should sit in meditation..." (Anonymous) – Matheus Bertelli (Pexels)
"The pose begins when..." (Baron Baptiste) – Alex Green (Pexels)
"Fill your bowl to the brim..." (Lao Tzu) – Christopher Burns (Unsplash)
"We show up, burn brightly..." (Rolf Gates) – Anastasia Pavlova (Pexels)
"Meditation is not evasion..." (Thich Nhat Hanh) – Jack Redgate (Pexels)
"Altogether, the idea of meditation..." (Chögyam Trungpa) – Andrew Gook (Unsplash)
"The mind is everything..." (Gautama Buddha) – Allan Mas (Pexels)
"If you begin to understand..." (Jiddu Krishnamurti) – Eberhard Grossgasteiger (Pexels)
"Peace comes from within..." (Gautama Buddha) – Stijn Dijkstra (Pexels)
"People are running, running..." (Paramahansa Yogananda) – Mohdi Bafande (Unsplash)
"That's life: Starting over..." (Sharon Salzberg) – Dziana Hasanbekava (Pexels)
"Imagine holding onto..." (Joseph Goldstein) – Henry Be (Unsplash)

INSIGHTS

INSIGHTS (SECTION COVER) – Tsvetoslav Hristov (Pexels)
At Your Limits, See What's Real – Taryn Elliott (Pexels)
Beginner's Mind – Pixabay (Pexels)
"When we don't know..." – Justyn Warner (Unsplash)
Being Teachable – Budgeron Bach (Pexels)
Comfortable Discomfort – Mikhail Nilov (Pexels)
"However we wish to take them..." – Jonathan Gallegos (Unsplash)
Get Clear – Fabio Comparelli (Unsplash)
"As the distractions blur..." – Jonathan Knepper (Unsplash)
Go Easy – Liza Summer (Pexels)
Living with Heart – Tobias Baur (Pexels)
Noting Life – Gianluca Grisenti (Pexels)
"The thing that keeps us..." – Oussema Rattazi (Unsplash)
Navigating Change – Anas Hinde (Pexels)
"All we can do is understand..." – Jon Tyson (Unsplash)
Practicing Integrity – Mikhail Nilov (Pexels)

START BY SITTING

START BY SITTING (SECTION COVER) – Light Wizzi (Pexels)
Introduction – Taryn Elliott (Pexels)
Day One – Tom Van Hoogstraten (Unsplash)
Day Two – Rachel Claire (Pexels)
Day Three – Rachel Claire (Pexels)
Day Four – Ekaterina Bolovtsova (Pexels)
Day Five – Uriel Mont (Pexels)
Day Six – Erik Mclean (Pexels)
Day Seven – Engin Akyurt (Unsplash)

ABOUT THE AUTHOR –   Josie Cipriano

"Everything that has a beginning..." (Jack Kornfield) – Kace Rodriguez (Unsplash)

BACK COVER

Pawel L. (Pexels)

YOGA

YOGA (SECTION COVER) – Taryn Elliott (Pexels)
TADASANA / MOUNTAIN POSE – cottonbro (Pexels)
VRKSASANA / TREE POSE – Josie Cipriano
ANUVITTASANA / STANDING BACKBEND POSE – Madison Lavern (Unsplash)
PARIVRTTA ARDHA PADMASANA / REVOLVED HALF LOTUS POSE – Dane Wetton (Unsplash)
URDHVA MUKHA SVANASANA / UPWARD FACING DOG POSE – GingerKitten (ShutterStock)
ADHO MUKHA SVANASANA / DOWNWARD FACING DOG POSE – koldunovaaa (Bigstock Photo)
ANJANEYASANA / LOW LUNGE / CRESCENT MOON POSE – Josie Cipriano
UTTANASANA / ACTIVE FORWARD FOLD / FORWARD BENDING POSE – Prostock-Studio (Bigstock Photo)
UTTHITA TRIKONASANA / TRIANGLE POSE – Mar Shani (Unsplash)
PASCHIMOTTANASANA / SEATED FORWARD BEND POSE – Benn McGuinness (Unsplash)

NATARAJASANA / KING DANCER POSE – Audrey Badin (Pexels)
URDHVA DHANURASANA / WHEEL / UPWARD FACING BOW POSE – Zachary Kyra-Derksen (Unsplash)
VIRABHADRASANA I / WARRIOR I POSE – Elina Fairytale (Pexels)
VIRABHADRASANA II / WARRIOR II POSE – Dragon Images (Bigstock Photo)
VIRABHADRASANA III / WARRIOR III POSE – Dmitriy Frantsev (Unsplash)
BALASANA / CHILD'S POSE – Balu Gaspar (Pexels)
PRASARITA PADOTTANASANA / WIDE-LEGGED FORWARD BEND POSE – Liveology Yoga Magazine (Unsplash)
UTTHITA HASTA PADANGUSTASANA / EXTENDED HAND-TO-TOE POSE – Chudakov_2 (Bigstock Photo)
SAVASANA / CORPSE POSE – Lola-Jane Genus

Sources

115   "The quieter you become, the more you can hear."   Dass, Ram. Be Here Now [enhanced edition]. HarperOne, 2010.

117   "Do your practice and all is coming."
Scott, John, and Shri K. Pattabhi Jois. Ashtanga Yoga: The Definitive Step-by-step Guide to Dynamic Yoga. Harmony Books, 2001.

119   "Fighting to preserve our mind...is only possible with the greatest of alertness."
Chwasan, Venerable. The Principle and Training of the Mind. Residence of the Prime Dharma Master Emeritus, 2012.

121   "In the untrained mind there is ceaseless movement, filled with plans, ideas, and memories. Seeing this previously unconscious stream of inner dialogue is for most people the first insight in [meditation] practice."   Goldstein, Joseph and Jack Kornfield. Seeking the Heart of Wisdom: The Path of Insight Meditation. Shambhala Publications, 2001.

123   "We have never stayed home long enough to experience the truth about ourselves."
Schiffmann, Erich. Yoga: The Spirit And Practice Of Moving Into Stillness. Simon and Schuster, 1996.

125   "The next message you need is always right where you are." [Unsourced]

127   "Everything happens for you, not to you".   Katie, Byron and Stephen Mitchell. A Mind at Home with Itself: How Asking Four Questions Can Free Your Mind, Open Your Heart, and Turn Your World Around. HarperCollins, 2018.

129   "The only way to live is by accepting each minute as an unrepeatable miracle."
Brach, Tara. Radical Acceptance: Embracing Your Life With the Heart of a Buddha. Bantam Books, 2003.

131   "Our actions almost always correspond to dispositions of mind. When I am impatient, traffic moves too slowly; when I am angry, others are irritating; when consumed and preoccupied with myself, other people only get in the way... This means that we don't need to wait around for the culture to change – the imbalances right in front of our eyes are laid out like freshly stretched canvases."
Stone, Michael. Yoga for a World Out of Balance: Teachings on Ethics and Social Action. Shambhala Publications, 2009.

133   "Your life doesn't get any better than your mind is: You might have wonderful friends, perfect health, a great career, and everything else you want, and you can still be miserable. The converse is also true: There are people who basically have nothing — who live in circumstances that you and I would do more or less anything to avoid — who are happier than we tend to be because of the character of their minds. Unfortunately, one glimpse of this truth is never enough. We have to be continually reminded of it."   Harris, Dan. Interview by Sam Harris. Taming the Mind, 17 Sept. 2014, https://www.samharris.org/blog/taming-the-mind. Accessed 27 Jan 2022.

135   "You are the sky - everything else, it's just the weather." [Unsourced]

137   "Rather than being your thoughts and emotions, be the awareness behind them."
Tolle, Eckhart. A New Earth: Awakening to Your Life's Purpose. Penguin Books, 2005.

139   "I believe that attention is the singular most important asset for anybody trying to achieve anything."   Vaynerchuk, Gary. "How to Get Your Business the Most Attention Possible in 2020." Game Changers Summit, 13 Dec 2019, Hotel at Avalon, Alpharetta, GA. Keynote Address.

141   "It is the power to focus the consciousness on a given spot, and hold it there. Attention is the first and indispensable step in all knowledge."
Patanjali. Yoga Sutras of Patanjali. Translated by Charles Johnston, The Quarterly Book Department, 1912.

143   "The real meditation is how you live your life."
Kabat-Zinn, Jon. Full Catastrophe Living: Using the Wisdom of Your Body and Mind to Face Stress, Pain, and Illness. Bantam Books, 1990.

145   "Yoga does not remove us from the reality or responsibilities of everyday life but rather places our feet firmly and resolutely in the practical ground of experience. We don't transcend our lives; we return to the life we left behind in the hopes of something better."
Farhi, Donna. Bringing Yoga to Life: The Everyday Practice of Enlightened Living. Harper Collins, 2003.

147   "Move a muscle, change a feeling." [Unsourced]

149 "Yoga has never been about the stretch; it's always been about the reach."
Corn, Seane. Revolution of the Soul: Awaken to Love Through Raw Truth, Radical Healing, and Conscious Action. Sounds True, 2019.

151 "Sometimes you need to sit lonely on a floor in a quiet room in order to hear your own voice and not let it drown in the noise of others."
Eriksson, Charlotte. You're Doing Just Fine. Broken Glass Records: Press & Distribution, 2015.

153 "If we feed ourselves noise on a regular basis, until we don't even recognize it as noise, how can we expect to quiet the mind?"
Strom, Max. A Life Worth Breathing: A Yoga Master's Handbook of Strength, Grace and Healing. Skyhorse Publishing, 2010.

155 "Endure both [the good and the bad], whichever arises." Gyatso, Geshe Kelsang. Universal Compassion: Inspiring Solutions for Difficult Times.
Tharpa Publications, 1988.

157 "Accept - then act. Whatever the present moment contains, accept it as if you had chosen it. Always work with it, not against it...This will miraculously transform your whole life." Tolle, Eckhart. The Power of Now: A Guide to Spiritual Enlightenment. New World Library, 2004.

159 "An intellectual mind that is unconnected to the heart is an uncultivated mind." Iyengar, BKS. Yoga: The Path to Holistic Health. DK, 2014.

161 "Love is the bridge between you and everything." [Unsourced]

163 "You should sit in meditation for twenty minutes a day – unless you're too busy; then you should sit for an hour." [Unsourced]

165 "The [pose] begins when you want to get out of it." Baptiste, Baron. Perfectly Imperfect: The Art and Soul of Yoga Practice. Hay House, 2016.

167 "Fill your bowl to the brim and it will spill. Keep sharpening your knife and it will blunt. Chase after money and security and your heart will never unclench. Care about people's approval and you will be their prisoner. Do your work, then step back. The only path to serenity."
Tzu, Lao. Tao Te Ching [a New English Version]. Translated by Stephen Mitchell, Harper Perennial, 1988.

169 "We show up, burn brightly in the moment, live passionately, and when the moment is over, when our work is done, we step back and let go."
Gates, Rolf, and Katrina Kenison. Meditations from the Mat: Daily Reflections on the Path of Yoga. Anchor Books, 2002.

171 "Meditation is not evasion; it is a serene encounter with reality."
Hanh, Thich Nhat. The Miracle of Mindfulness: An Introduction to the Practice of Meditation. Translated by Mobi Ho, Beacon Press, 1975.

173 "Altogether, the idea of meditation is not to create states of ecstasy or absorption, but to experience being." Trungpa, Chögyam. The Path of Individual
Liberation: The Profound Treasury of the Ocean of Dharma, Volume One, compiled and edited by Judith L. Lief, Shambhala Publications, 2014.

175 "The mind is everything. What you think you become." [Unsourced]

177 "If you begin to understand what you are without trying to change it, then what you are undergoes a transformation."
Krishnamurti, Jiddu. The Book of Life: Daily Meditations with Krishnamurti. HarperCollins, 1995.

179 "Peace comes from within. Do not seek it without." [Unsourced]

181 "People are running, running, but there is no place in the world to which they can flee to escape themselves. Ultimately, each one must face himself."
Yogananda, Paramahansa. The Divine Romance: Collected Talks & Essays on Realizing God in Daily Life. Self Realization Fellowship, 1987.

183 "That's life: Starting over, one breath at a time." Salzberg, Sharon. Real Happiness: The Power of Meditation, a 28-Day Program. Workman Publishing, 2011.

185 "Imagine holding on to a hot burning coal. You would not fear letting go of it. In fact, once you noticed that you were holding on, you would probably drop it quickly. But we often do not recognize how we hold on to suffering. It seems to hold on to us. This is our practice: becoming aware of how suffering arises in our mind and of how we become identified with it, and learning to let it go. We learn through simple and direct observation, seeing the process over and over again until we understand." Goldstein, Joseph. Insight Meditation: A Psychology of Freedom. Shambhala Publications, 1993.

246 "Everything that has a beginning, has an ending. Make your peace with that and all will be well."
Kornfield, Jack. Buddah's Little Instruction Book. Bantam Books, 1994.

Acknowledgments

I extend primary gratitude to my very first yoga teacher, only ever known as 'Phil', who took a too-busy A-type and (gently, eccentrically, authentically) sparked something in her that would profoundly change the course of her life.

To the staff and karma yogis at Yasodhara Ashram in Kootenay Bay, thank you for your most gracious and memorable introduction to the concepts herein.

Unending thanks to every single soul—master teacher, instructor, staff, student—who walked through the doors at what was once Semperviva Yoga Studios in Vancouver, Canada.

To Gloria Latham, owner and manager of these studios and master teacher in her own right, I am so grateful to have been part of your team and to have been privy to your wisdom and insight, on and off the mat. To the men and women who became my friends and family within those walls, you are in every page of this book.

Swamis Tatwarupananda Saraswati, Nivedanananda Saraswati and Govindanada Saraswati, my dearest swami-ji, I learned more about consciousness and what is Real in one month with you than in decades of books, practice and study.

To the best book-team an author could ask for—Akosua (Jackie) Brown, Erika Arcos and Maxine Wray. Thank you so much for helping make this dream of mine a reality.

To those in my *doing-life-with-me* circles, I am forever thankful:

My parents and brother for being the ones who've known, seen and guided me for longer than anyone on the planet. *Los quiero con todo mi corazón, mis amigos del alma.* The Hills, for remaining my family throughout the storms. Los Candia, los Pizzorno, los Maggi, los De Romaña—*familia extensa, siempre parte mía.*

Nadine Lobinowich, Jenne Todd, Karen Williams Skelton, Kim Candia—my life sisters. Bronwyn Storoschuk, Mallory Harris, Keara Taylor, Erin Valente, Laura Von Hagen, Heather Robinson, Tamara Kung, Michelle McKee, Alvin Campaña, Rossana Cogorno—from our first school days until forever. Kerri King, for being so generous with your time and insights on my manuscript. Karen Beal, for guiding and mentoring me far beyond clinical practice.

My baby girl, River Mae, who is about the wisest soul I've ever known and who inspires me to always do better.

And to Mother Nature. The original inspiration.
Thank you, thank you, thank you.

About the Author

Dr. Ana Candia, ND is a yoga & mindfulness mentor, wellness leader & Naturopathic Doctor.

Prior to her naturopathic medical training, Dr. Candia interspersed years of formal study in Human Biology, Globalization and Education with extended periods of international work and volunteerism with Naturopaths Without Borders, Natural Doctors International as well as Feed the Children.

Dr. Candia is a licensed yoga instructor and has developed and taught courses in key health foundations. She is a second generation Argentine-Canadian, a proud mother of one, and above all else, a student of Nature.

She lives, breathes and practices in Durham, Ontario.

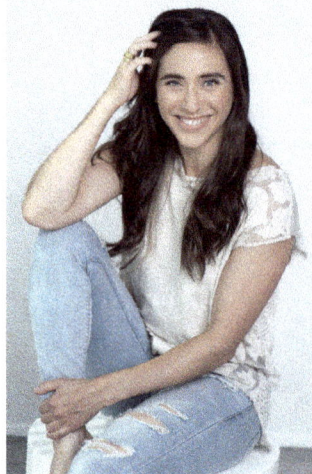

www.ingramcontent.com/pod-product-compliance
Lightning Source LLC
Chambersburg PA
CBHW040835300326
41914CB00061B/1391